Health Policy

This important new textbook provides comparative and critical analysis of health care policy from high-income countries in Europe to low-income developing countries in the Global South.

It integrates conceptual themes drawn from the fields of sociology, policy analysis, and political science to offer a unique combination of theory, historical background, and wider social commentary. The book is divided into three sections:

- Section I establishes the conceptual basis for the analysis of the health policymaking process, including implementation.
- Section II provides an introduction to the key elements of conducting a comparative health system's analysis, including chapters that provide examples of performance analysis in both high- and low-income developing countries.
- Section III examines key challenges now facing health policy-makers that include long-term social care provision, widening the scope of public health to address social inequalities in health outcome, the integration of genomic medicine within a health care system, and the establishment of an effective national pharmaceutical policy.

Each chapter includes case studies, historical-institutional contexts, and summaries of key health policies. Detailed and clearly written, it is the ideal text for health and social science students in this expanding area of analysis.

Iain Crinson has been teaching, researching, and publishing in the field of the sociology of health and health policy for over three decades. For much of this time, he has been based at St Georges, University of London.

Health Policy

Critical and Comparative Perspectives

Iain Crinson

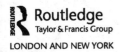
Routledge
Taylor & Francis Group

LONDON AND NEW YORK

Designed cover image: Getty

First published 2025
by Routledge
4 Park Square, Milton Park, Abingdon, Oxon OX14 4RN

and by Routledge
605 Third Avenue, New York, NY 10158

Routledge is an imprint of the Taylor & Francis Group, an informa business

© 2025 Iain Crinson

The right of Iain Crinson to be identified as author of this work has been asserted in accordance with sections 77 and 78 of the Copyright, Designs and Patents Act 1988.

British Library Cataloguing-in-Publication Data
A catalogue record for this book is available from the British Library

ISBN: 978-1-032-91621-7 (hbk)
ISBN: 978-1-032-34576-5 (pbk)
ISBN: 978-1-003-56424-9 (ebk)

DOI: 10.4324/9781003564249

Typeset in Sabon
by KnowledgeWorks Global Ltd.

Contents

CONTENTS

Figures and tables

Figures

Tables

Acknowledgements

Without the support of my partner Lorna, and my sons Elliott and Miles, this book might well have taken even longer to research, write, and finally complete.

General introduction

This textbook is concerned to develop an integrated analysis of health policy and health systems. The use of the term 'integrated' is not a throwaway phrase; it reflects an underpinning thread that runs throughout the structure of this book that embraces a range of academic disciplinary approaches and theoretical perspectives. The intended audience includes final year undergraduates as well as post-graduates who are undertaking modules in the field of health policy studies, health care management, and comparative studies of public policy. It will also be of interest to professional practitioners in the field of health and social care.

The book itself is divided into three analytically distinct but integrated domains of health policy analysis. The first section is intended to provide the conceptual tools of public policy and health system analysis. In doing so, it draws on a critical reading of the established health policy literature, from an assessment of the interventionist health and welfare role of the state, to the standard models of the policy-making process, then to an appraisal of health system governance and its constituents, then onto a critique of the typologies of funding and financing health care.

The second section is concerned with comparative health system analysis. Engaging in the process of comparing the performance and institutional histories of health care systems is a relatively recent development in the health policy field. Where once health systems were studied in isolation from one another, often with elements of national bias, the expansion in digitalised health information systems has facilitated ready access to comparative performance data. This development has drawn attention to the fact that there are frequently more commonalities than differences across health systems. This section will provide an introduction to the analytical frameworks that are drawn upon in conducting a systematic comparative analysis. It then provides two examples of comparative systems analysis. One focuses on health systems in two high-income countries, Germany and the UK, and the second, two health systems in low-income developing countries, Ghana and Kenya.

The final section of the book moves onto a detailed assessment of three contrasting, but linked challenges that health care systems in high-income countries have conspicuously failed to come to terms with over the past two decades. The first is the issue of ageing populations and a concordant rising demand for long-term social care provision. The second challenge is that of widening the scope of public health provision, an area of intervention that has frequently been marginalised yet has the potential to play a crucial role in addressing the widening gap in social inequalities in health outcome. The third challenge is that of the integration of genomic medicine into the mainstream

DOI: 10.4324/9781003564249-1

of health care system, linked to a critical assessment of the role of 'Big Pharma' and the attempt by the UK government to develop a 'pharmaceutical policy'.

****

Use of Endnotes: Endnotes are utilised throughout the book to draw attention to additional details that may be of interest for wider social analysis. Additionally, the integrative approach adopted within this book necessarily means that the same conceptual frames of analysis appear at various points across the text in reference to different aspects of health policy and health systems. In order to avoid repetition, endnotes are used to guide the reader to where the substantive discussion of that concept sits within the book.

Conceptualising and Contextualising Health Policy

Introduction to Section I

The objective of this first section is to establish the basis for the interdisciplinary approach that is a key feature of this book. That is, the bringing together of a range of analytical perspectives drawn from the sociology of organisations, political science, economics, and historical institutionalism applied to the analysis of health policy and health systems. On this point, it should also be noted at that a distinction is often drawn within the literature between the use of the terms 'health policy', 'health care policy', and 'health care politics' (Blank et al:2018;2). This is not purely a semantic distinction, as each of these appellations does indeed designate distinct fields of research. 'Health policy' examines in broad terms the courses of action proposed and implemented by governments that impact on the health outcomes of a population. Health policy analysis necessarily overlaps with other areas of governmental public policy, in particular social welfare policies as well as State fiscal policy. 'Health care policy' is a more focused designation that assesses the courses of action associated with the funding and provision of primary and secondary care services within a given health care system such as the National Health Service (NHS). Finally, the designation 'health care politics' includes the analysis of the role and interactions of political actors and organisations (both internal and external to state structures) involved in the determination of health policy objectives and priorities in a given system. This book will seek to embrace and integrate all three fields of analysis.

Reference

Blank, R, Burau, V and Kuhlmann, E (2018) *Comparative Health Policy* (5th Ed). Basingstoke. Palgrave.

DOI: 10.4324/9781003564249-2

Globalisation and the changing role of the state

Theorising the role of the state

Any critical assessment of the role of the state in modern capitalist economies necessarily reflects the epistemological pre-assumptions of policy analysts. It is often difficult to maintain empirical objectivity in the contested ideological battleground that constitutes the field of state economic, social, and health policy. On this basis, it is appropriate to delineate the main theoretical positions that have informed the competing explanations of the historical role played by the state in modern societies.

The first of these perspectives is known as *Classic Pluralism*. Pluralism conceives the state as essentially a neutral instrument that enacts the will of the people, represented by political parties, within participatory democratic societies. Elected governments are seen as having the power and authority to enact change and alter the direction and scope of policy by virtue of their democratic mandate, that is, public policy outcomes are reflective of the balance of forces and social divisions in society registered, but not mediated, by government in the 'public interest' (Pierson:1996;73–74).

The second approach is known as *Elite theory* and is traditionally linked with populist politics. The role of the state is conceived as primarily one of maintaining or 'legitimising' the social and economic interests of powerful groups within society. In its classic form, Elite theory asserts that the social groups who achieve their position of power in a given political system do so solely by virtue of their control over key resources. In modern societies this power manifests as control over economic resources, but can also include knowledge and expertise, as well as traditional forms of high social status or charisma. A particularly radical version of Elite theory appears in the work of the eminent American sociologist, C. Wright Mills (1956). Writing in the mid-1950s, Wright-Mills identified three hegemonic institutions in American society (the military, major industrial corporations, and the US government itself), seen as holding the 'pivotal positions' within that society. The individuals holding the top positions within these institutions at any given time were seen as having similar sets of social and economic interests and so engaged in mutually supportive activities that together constituted a national 'power elite'. From this perspective, the formation of state policy should be assessed in terms of which major institutions, as well as social groups, are the beneficiaries of said policy and which are not.

A third perspective is known as *Neoliberalism* and is particularly associated with the political economic theories of Friedrich Hayek. It combines explanation with prescription, together with a post-1970's libertarian disillusionment with the interventionist role of the social democratic state. The latter being seen as, 'an increasingly domineering

DOI: 10.4324/9781003564249-3

and malign influence imposing itself upon society' (Pierson:1996;80). Hayek's political ideology was influenced by traditional liberal economics (hence 'neo-liberalism') that dated as far back as Adam Smith's *Wealth of Nations* (2004) published in 1776. It was Adam Smith who contended that market forces should be always be given free rein to maximise the economies of self-interest. In principle, neoliberalism is opposed to state intervention on the grounds that it distorts the 'natural' self-interested equilibrium of the market. The state is also seen engaging in activities that serve to perpetuate its own institutional interests over that of individuals. In practice though, neoliberals often arrive at a compromise position vis-a-vis the interventionary role of the national state. This is an acceptance that some level of intervention is required to maintain economic and social infrastructure so as to ensure the efficient flow of goods and services. The caveat is that the levying of taxes, necessary to generate state revenue to fund even minimal interventions, is seen as subverting individual enterprise and autonomy. The apparent contradiction between neoliberal principles and practice frequently plays out in the plays-formation process of right-leaning governments that seek to determine what should be the minimum required of the state in providing a collective social and health safety net for the population.

The fourth perspective is known as *Political Economy* and is associated with, but not exclusive to, Marxist theories of the state. The understanding of the function and structure of the state is that it is neither fixed nor separate from wider economic processes. The role of the state is seen as tied into the wider requirements and interests of the nation[1] within a globalised capitalist economic system. This understanding emphasises the ways in which global economic financial crises directly impact on the functioning of the national state, while also emphasising the role played by the state as the major source of legitimation for that economic system. This process of legitimation extends to restraining and ameliorating the worst social excesses or 'external effects' of the capitalist economic market system. The national state is seen as achieving this requirement through the establishment of regulatory institutions that involve the imposition of legal and social controls, as well as the provision of health and welfare rights for citizens. But there are clear limits to the ability of a national state, drawing on its power and authority, to intervene in order to maintain social and economic stability: '(S)tate action can never be aware of or even guess, let alone implement or enforce everything that could be considered system-compatible intervention' (Dörre et al:2015;113[2]). This position would explicitly contend the oft-cited but frequently historically de-contextualised quotation from Marx's 'Communist Manifesto' published in 1848, that the state is simply an 'executive committee' for managing the 'common affairs of the bourgeoisie' (or capitalist class).

The establishment of the post-war welfare state
The establishment of 'universal social welfare' services provided as a right for all citizens in the immediate aftermath of the Second World War represented a significant historical expansion of the interventionist role of the national state, not only in Britain but in many other Western European countries, as well as Australasia; with the USA being the notable outlier. This provision of public services generally included universal health care, full-time education up to the age of 15, as well as financial support for citizens in the form of social protection or 'social security' What subsequently became termed the 'welfare state' represented a significant collectivist undertaking that reflected two

mutually inclusive goals, one of which could be described as *realist* or pragmatic and the other *idealist*. The pragmatic goal in constructing new state health and welfare institutions was to consolidate the solidarity and social cohesion that had been the experience of the majority of the population in these countries during the Second World War, despite the privations and personal sacrifices that had to be made. The realist aspect of state welfarism was ensuring that this ambitious project was fiscally sustainable following the near bankrupt financial situation that all countries in Europe found themselves in following the end of that war, whether or not that country could be described as 'victorious' or as 'vanquished'.

In the case of the UK, this idealism was reflected in the reception accorded the Beveridge[3] Report (1942) that was published in the middle of the Second World War, when victory over Nazi Germany was not at all certain. This report was an official investigation into the pre-war system of social insurance and welfare, but on the back of this analysis the report proposed a radically new structure for state welfarism with the goal of defeating the 'five giant evils' of want, disease, ignorance, squalor and idleness. The Beveridge Report not only proposed that a post-war government establish a system of social protection for all, but even more radically, recommended the 'setting up of a comprehensive medical service for every citizen, covering all treatment and every form of disability under the supervision of the Health Departments' (Beveridge Report:1942;para 106). The realist aspects of the Beveridge Report lay in the understanding that if the state took on the funding and provision of health care, social protection, housing, and pensions, then this would also serve to increase the productivity of workers and the competitiveness of British industry. Establishing a state funded welfare regime it was assumed would result in healthier, wealthier, more motivated, and therefore more productive workers and increase the demand for more consumable British manufactured products.

This state interventionist model was subsequently termed the 'Keynesian political-economic institutional system', as it was seen to reflect the prescriptions of the eminent 'anti-free market' economist John Maynard Keynes. This 'social market' approach was adopted and refined by the Christian Democratic government in post-war West Germany that was subsequently termed 'Rhine' or 'Rhenish' capitalism. The West German 'social market' was characterised by a central banking system that facilitated more effective financing of industry. Close economic ties were forged between the central bank, the financial ministries, and large manufacturing companies where an equal balance of power was constructed between shareholders and management. In order to bring the organised working class on-side and ensure industrial harmony, a 'social partnership' was built between the trade unions and employers (known as 'corporatism'). These new institutionalised corporatist structures were consolidated alongside the introduction of a series of comprehensive reforms to the system of social security and health care. However, the pre-war Social Insurance model of employee and employer contributions was to remain and indeed continues to the present day in a now unified Germany.[4] The mixture of business realism combined with greater institutionalised participatory rights for workers and their trade unions was deemed essential for the demands of post-war reconstruction. This mixture of idealism and realism that underpinned the building of a social and political consensus in Britain was also a characteristic feature of state policy in the majority of post-war Western European nations.

The prevailing view within policy analysis in the post-war period was that the expansive interventionary role for the national state constituted a key dimension of what was then regarded as a 'progressive' stage of capitalism. Progress was seen as constituted by the mixed 'social market economy' alongside the provision of state welfare benefits and health care, together with the development of new national 'collectivist' forms of economic planning. The broad agreement was that these developments could mitigate the worst excesses and outcomes of the capitalist system of production and distribution. The national state was therefore seen as taking on a mediating role, balancing the requirements of profitability against the need for social integration and relative distributive equity.

In Britain, the social market model never became as firmly institutionalised within the fabric of the economy as was the case in West Germany. However, the new welfare regime in Britain including the National Health Service (NHS) was arguably more ambitious in scope than the social health insurance model retained in Germany. In Sweden, a neutral nation during the war, a modern welfare state had begun to emerge in the late 1930s and expanded in the post-war period. While in France, a new system of social protection was established in 1946, this enshrined the right to a minimum standard of living regardless of the ability to contribute. However, it took rather longer to establish the principle of universal health care in France (not until 1999). Similar welfare state systems also emerged in the Benelux countries. In Southern Europe, the decimation of economic infrastructure and violent confrontation between political parties of the right and Left following the end of the war (as well as the continuity of authoritarian regimes in both Spain and Portugal) made it much more difficult to initially implement the social market model and social protection and universal health care policies found elsewhere. But eventually here too, welfare state models were firmly established by the late 1970s.

Fiscal crises and the sustainability of health and welfare systems

To study the formation and development of health policy and health care systems is also to recognise the economic, fiscal, and social 'crises' that served to constrain the interventionist role of the nation state towards the end of the twentieth century; noting that, 'the parallels and interactions among capitalist countries far outweigh their institutional and economic differences' (Streek:2017;lx). 'Crisis theory' that emerged in the early 1970s is a critique of the inevitability of a progressive state social welfarism. Crisis theory was a realist response to the optimism that had been associated with the 'golden years' of post-war reconstruction and the development of 'welfare states'. Specifically, the use of the term 'crisis' focused attention on the social and cultural role played by the state in 'legitimating' the accumulation of capital (profits). While Crisis theory itself frequently evoked Lenin's famous dictum set out in 1917 in his 'State and Revolution' (Lenin:1976) where he asserted that the democratic state always acts as 'the best possible political shell for capitalism'. In other words, there could be no illusions as to the long-term sustainability of post-war state welfarism, and the 'progressive values' manifest in the social market model. By the end of the 1970s, this critique appeared to be borne out by the re-emergence in the political and economic mainstream of the ideology of economic liberalism and free markets.

The increasingly globalised nature of the post-war system of capitalist production and distribution has led to much greater uncertainty in developing national macroeconomic policy (regulating the circulation of credit and debit in the financial system) and fiscal policy (taxing and spending). The limits to the autonomy of the state in determining the direction of economic and political policy was eventually to put at risk the post-war 'social contract' that guaranteed the basic health care and welfare needs of all citizens. Over the past 50 years (that is, since the mid-1970s), while the economies of Western countries have continued to grow, this has been at a much slower rate than historically was the case. This assessment takes into consideration those periods such as the mid to late 1990s, where high rates of growth were achieved but not sustained over the long-term. As a consequence, national governments have to increasingly borrow on the international financial markets to fund their existing health and welfare commitments, which in turn has led to a rise in overall national debt in many of these high-income countries.

The long-term costs of the Second World War meant that even as late as 1960, Britain continued to experience particularly high levels of public debt. However, the general trend in the majority of high-income countries (HIC's) with some exceptions as represented in Figure 1.1 shows that by the late 1970s, average national debt coalesced somewhere between 20% and 40% of GDP. This reflected the high growth rate experienced by these economies from the 1950s up until the early 1970s, but which ended abruptly following the significant hike in energy prices during the 'Oil crises' of 1973. This was one of several national and international factors that together contributed to fiscal crisis, economic slowdown, rising unemployment levels, and increasing levels of public debt.

The fact that public expenditure continued to increase in these HIC's up until the mid-1990 while fiscal deficit widened does not mean that spending on health and welfare can be attributed to the demands of an 'insatiable electorates', as was claimed by

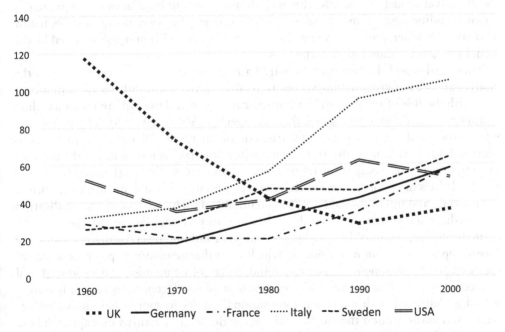

Figure 1.1 Government debt as percentage (%) of GDP post-war timeline of selected high-income countries (Adapted from IMF (2022)).

neoliberal commentators at the time. On the contrary, as Wolfgang Streek has argued, there is much to be said for a functionalist view of a continued increase in state spending during a period of fiscal crises as serving the best long-term interests of capital. State public service spending, 'expressed a growing need for public investment and curative measures to accompany capitalist development – measures that repaired the damage caused by capital accumulation as well as creating the conditions for further growth' (Streek:2017;68). Yet the position that sustaining the level of public spending was crucial to the stimulation of a demand-side led economy was to be set aside over the following decades with the increasing prominence of neo-liberal thinking in government policy.

In contrast to the post-war political consensus that saw the primary role of the state as guaranteeing the rights of citizens to health and welfare in a social market, the neoliberal political and economic position was that the public were 'consumers', whose choices were best exercised by buying and selling in an unfettered competitive marketplace. The notion of the 'invisible hand', first given prominence in Adam Smith's (1759) *laissez-faire* economic philosophy, was re-invoked in the contention that the economic marketplace delivered benefits that could never be achieved by state planning. This perspective represented a particular interpretation of a linked series of economic and social processes manifest from the late 1970s. These included the exponential rise in mass consumerism that was facilitated by the increasingly ready availability of cheap personal credit, a process made possible by national government's inflating of the national money supply. Together, these developments can be seen as reflecting a 'cultural acceptance of market-adjusted and market-driven ways of life' (Streek:2017;3–4). This popular 'acceptance' appeared to be manifest in the election to power of a series of right wing market-orientated governments committed to limiting or curtailing the social market model. In the UK, this new thinking was influential in the approach to public spending adopted by the newly elected Conservative government in 1979, led by Margaret Thatcher, and a few years later with the 'Voodoo Economics'[5] adopted by the Ronald Regan administration in the USA.

These real-world developments required a re-appraisal of Crisis theory, and so the analytical focus of critical analysis began to shift in the late 1980s away from a concern with the role of the state in legitimising capitalism and towards an understanding of capital as 'an apparatus rather than an agency' (Streek:2017;18). The new focus was on the implications for state welfarism of an emerging global process that was to become known as 'financialisation'. Financialisation has been defined as 'the increasing importance of financial markets, financial motives, financial institutions and financial elites in the operations of the economy and its governing institutions, both at the national and international levels' (Epstein:2001;1). The process of financialisation was predicated on a renewed confidence in the ability of international markets to self-regulate and underpinned by neoliberal economic thinking. It served to undermine the classic supply-side economic model in which capital accumulation (profit generation) followed from investment in the stocks and shares of companies that produced and sold commodities. A new demand-led economic model reflected an increasingly unregulated global market that enabled international banks to more easily move investments and loans around the world, looking for the highest returns on capital. These were also the financial opportunities that frequently carried the highest risk. Banks began to internationalise and develop new financial products such as syndicated loans and credit derivatives that enabled them to shift risk management activities off their portfolio balance sheets. Derivatives made it easier for banks to decouple the risk profile from their origination business. By 2007, the worldwide derivative assets of international banks had increased from about 1 trillion US Dollars in 1998 to 17 trillion US Dollars at its peak (McCauley et al:2021). These unrestricted developments significantly contributed to the boom in cheap credit enabling dramatic increases in global market demand for goods and services in the 1990s and up to 2008.

Over and above national differences and questions of sovereignty, the combined process of globalisation and financialisation appeared to give weight to the case made by neoliberal politicians that public services should be 'modernised' in order to take advantage of this 'new order' of things. 'Modernisation' being the umbrella term used to justify this policy shift towards market 'reforms' within public services, one which emphasised 'efficiency', 'competitiveness', and cost-reduction strategies over service user needs and patient equity. In the UK, 'modernisation' became the mantra for a radical restructuring of the NHS proposed and partially enacted by the Conservative government led by Margaret Thatcher in 1989. The concept continued to retain its prominence a decade later in the health service reforms introduced by Tony Blair's 'New Labour' government. While the latter was ostensibly committed to reducing the social gap in health inequalities, at the same time it did little to resist the growing macroeconomic pressure to reduce public spending. Many of these pressures emanated from the World Trade Organisation (WTO) which in 1995 had replaced the General Agreement on Tariffs and Trade – GATT. WTO rules now required that public services be subject to the same rules of competition that was previously restricted to the trading of goods. In the UK, and throughout the European Union, public services including health care were now subject to the global process of market reform or 'marketisation'. Marketisation was the term used to describe the restructuring of the regulatory and legal environment for the provision of public services that opened-up the possibilities for profit-making in delivering public services. This process of marketisation combined with the new 'financialised' economic environment began to have a direct impact on future public investment decision-making strategy in relation to health and welfare systems (Karwowski:2019).[6]

In the UK, one of the better-known examples of what was to became known as 'public-private partnerships' that arose from a marketised public service environment, was the Private Finance Initiative (PFI). This was, and remains (albeit downscaled from 2018) a strategy to encourage private capital to invest in a hospital building programme for the NHS. The programme was initially launched in 1992, but only really expanded in scope during the period of the New Labour government (1997–2010). PFI enabled the government to shift some of the cost and therefore responsibility for delivering public services, onto private capital. During this period when cheap credit was readily available, commercial companies were able to borrow money with the sole aim of acquiring valuable state assets. PFI guaranteed these companies long-term income from the rents that they charged for the use of privately financed facilities that included new hospitals, health centres as well as schools and other public services. These interlinked processes (financialisation, marketisation, and privatisation) have had a long-term impact in shifting the way in which the institutional assets of the state, including schools, hospitals, playing fields, and libraries were now to be assessed, now primarily in terms of their capital value (as property and land) rather than 'public goods'.

The impact of the 2007 banking crises on state health and welfare spending

The availability of cheap credit and the naïve assumptions about the workings of the global financial system that underpinned it was severely undermined following the near collapse of the international banking system in 2007. Economic crisis followed an accumulation of defaulted loans across the globe, but particularly within the USA, where there was an implosion of the 'sub-prime' market for home mortgages. The investment exposures of banks in this highly risky market were just too great and this led onto a generalised collapse in the confidence of the global financial markets, and with it the cheap credit that national economic growth strategies had become reliant upon. National economic stagnation in a majority of countries across the globe now followed the cutting-off of credit flows to both the public and private employment sectors. This process fed into rising national budgetary deficits, and still further increases in the level of public debt.

By 2008, governments were being forced into the position of acting as 'lifeboats' of last resort to prop-up national banking systems covering their losses through the buying back of government bonds[7] that had previously been invested in by these very same banks. Both in the UK and the Eurozone (as directed by the European Central Bank) this involved a process known as Quantitative Easing(QE), defined as large-scale purchases of financial assets in return for central bank reserves.[8] In the UK the purchasing of these bonds was enabled though a process of 'printing' electronic money and drawn upon by the Asset Purchase Facility (APF), a legally separate entity created for just this purpose run by the Bank of Enland with indemnity assurances from the Treatury (Breedon et al:2012). By 2009, the UK government net borrowing requirement was approximately £150 billion, double the estimates that had initially been forecast. This was a direct consequence of the government's financial rescue package which included a £37 billion recapitalisation for the main UK banks, and £21 billion to the Bank of England to assist in the refinancing of the financial services sector (IFS:2009). The evidence from a series of quantitative studies that have been published subsequently has found, 'a positive correlation between the size of a country's financial sector and the scale of new debt taken on in the wake of the crises' (Streek:2017;49).

Over the following decade, the UK government adopted a mixture of fiscal and monetary measures, not always in synch, in an attempt to further resuscitate the banking and financial sector and so reduce the high level of public debt. But these fiscal interventions were ultimately at the cost of reducing real terms state spending on health and welfare services and provision. Monetary policy in the UK has been strictly the province of the Bank of England since 1997, while fiscal policy is the responsibility of the government (specifically, the UK Treasury). Yet these events clearly demonstrated how both are inextricably linked. Alongside these monetary interventions, the UK Treasury initiated a fiscal policy that embraced a series of 'austerity budgets' that set limits on government spending and were manifest in real terms reductions in state health and welfare expenditure. This fiscal policy remained in place until the COVID-19 pandemic forced a dramatic increase in government spending, with massive injections of cash for new public health measures, as well as compensation for businesses who lost income arising from the national isolation strategy.

The post-2007 banking collapse directly contributed to a widening in the fiscal gap or 'fiscal balance', calculated as total government revenues minus total government expenditures. Fiscal balance is one of several internationally agreed concepts, definitions, classifications, and rules for national accounting that are utilised within the OECD National Accounts Statistics database (OECD:2021). This database is the primary source of the statistics presented in Figure 1.2 and shows that in the six selected high-income countries, all with extensive state managed health care and welfare systems, fiscal balance as a percentage of Gross Domestic Product[9] (GDP) begin to narrow over the course of 12 years of public spending austerity. Prior to the COVID-19 pandemic and the concomitant rise in government expenditure combined with the reductions in revenue associated with business losses and personal income reductions, the fiscal balance in OECD countries reached an average of −3.2% of GDP in 2019. Over the long-term economic cycle, the attempt by these governments to achieve fiscal balance since the 2007 crises had been spectacularly unsuccessful.

As Wolfgang Streek has argued; '(S)ince 2008, governments have had little or no idea how to clear away the debris of the financial crisis and recreate some kind of order

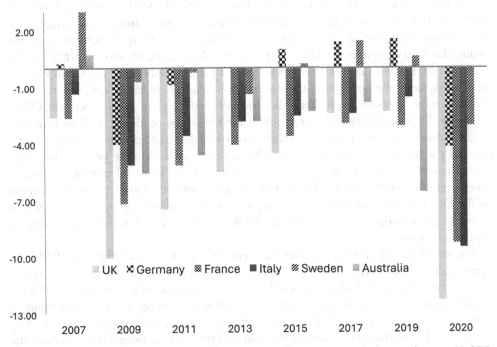

Figure 1.2 The 'Fiscal Gap' post-2007 total government revenues minus total expenditure as % GDP (Adapted from OECD (2021))

– a task that certainly cannot be privatized. In the measures taken by governments and central banks to save the private banking system, the distinction between public and private money has become increasing irrelevant. Today it is virtually impossible to tell where the state ends and the market begins, and whether governments have been nationalizing banks, or banks have been privatizing the state' (2017;40). The economic slowdown that following the 2007 banking crises has negatively impacted on the ability of national states to sustain previous levels of public expenditure sufficient to meet the ever-expanding health and social needs of their populations. The potential scope for increases in personal taxation alone in order to increase public spending is limited, with average real wages in decline across high-income countries. In the UK in the period from 1970 to 2007, real term wages grew by an average 33 per cent, but this fell to below zero in the decade of 2010–20 (Resolution Foundation:2022).

Concluding comments: democracy, welfarism, and the markets

The power of the global financial markets to effectively curtail the spending decisions of democratically elected governments is well illustrated in the classic story told by Bob Woodward of the *Washington Post* about Bill Clinton[10] when he first came into office in 1993. Clinton was informed that if he went ahead and carried out the full programme of spending commitments that had formed the main plank of his successful electoral campaign, then the US central bank, the Federal Reserve, would raise US interest rates to protect the value of government bonds even if it meant an increased risk of recession. Clinton's reported response was: 'You mean to tell me that the success of the programme and my re-election hinges on the Federal Reserve and a bunch of f****** bond traders?' (Woodward:1994).Whether or not, Clinton was actually that naïve about the power of the markets is questionable, but their capacity to limit the options for intervention of even the most powerful democratically elected official in the world is not. In 2010, one of the first actions of George Osbourne, the Chancellor of the Exchequer of the newly elected Conservative government in the UK, was to establish within the Treasury, an in-house but formally independent public body, the Office for Budget Responsibility (OBR) to provide advice on the economic and fiscal impact of government spending policies. So that effectively, the markets were not only 'legally encased via law and regulation, but psychically encased within the political imagination' (Davies:2022;3). Both examples demonstrate how the financial markets are able to exert leverage over the fiscal policies of elected governments. This in turn sets limits to public spending, particularly spending on state health and welfare programmes which is frequently presented as constraining economic growth, and thus limiting returns for capital investment.

The crises in public finances that has been ever present since the late 1970s has been described by Streek (2017) as the transition from a 'tax state' to a 'debt state', and this transition is linked to the neoliberal transformation of post-war social market welfare capitalism. To this extent, Streek identifies the emergence of, 'a new stage in the relationship between capitalism and democracy, as the state subjects itself and its activity to the control of creditors in the shape of markets … alongside the democratic control of the state by its citizenry, with the possibility of overlaying it, or even eliminating it altogether' (Streek:2017;78). While global financial creditors, 'cannot vote out a government that is not to their liking; they can, however, sell off their existing bonds or refrain from participating in a new auction of public debt' (Streek:2017;81). This dynamic played out, possibly in ways not even anticipated by Wolfgang Streek, when in October 2022, the UK Conservative Prime Minister, Liz Truss was forced to resign after six weeks in power and a new government was constituted. This followed on from her government's failure to get support from the financial markets to endorse a popularist tax-cutting budget. The markets lacked confidence in the ability of Truss's government to service any increase in debts and was concerned about any fiscal easing that would lead on to higher interest rates. The Bank of England was then forced into a position where it had to attempt to regain financial market confidence through a spree of buying back government bonds, but with little avail. Whatever the merits of the UK government's attempt to develop a supply-side led growth in the economy, and these were few, this was nevertheless a policy that emanated from a democratically elected government. The unelected financial markets rejection of the economic strategy set out by the British government in 2022 led directly to the replacement of a Prime Minister and complete reversal of the main planks of the proposed national economic budget.

The global economic and financial developments that have been described in this chapter clearly demonstrate limits to the power of the national state in determining the direction and scope of public health and welfare policies. Yet, this is to be balanced against a continuing popular democratic support for universal state health and welfare provision. The necessity of massive state intervention to effectively manage the impact of COVID-19 pandemic crises has only reinforced the view that the infrastructural role played by the state remains essential and cannot be left to the vagaries of the market.

Notes

1 Interrogating the construct of the 'nation' and what constitutes the 'national interest' is a matter of concern that goes beyond the scope of this text. Suffice to state at this point that for 'nation' we cannot simply read territorial or sovereign homogeneity where the application of the term 'nation state' is much more accurate. The notion of the 'nation' remains contentious not just in political and economic terms, but also sociologically as well as culturally.
2 This account draws heavily on the work of the German social-political scientist, Claus Offe.
3 William Beveridge was an economist and former director of the London School of Economics who was appointed as an advisor to the wartime coalition government, initially to advise on manpower planning but, in 1942, was asked to survey the exiting system of social insurance and make recommendations with the view to post-war reform. His subsequent report was to shape the future direction of welfare provision in Britain.
4 Discussed at length in Chapter 7.
5 This term was actually coined by George Bush Senior when he unsuccessfully challenged Regan to be the Republican Party candidate for the US Election of 1980.
6 The implications of these process in relation to the organisation and governance of health care systems are discussed in detail in Chapter 3.
7 Bonds are securities that pay a fixed rate of return over a long-term period until maturity, they are bought by banks and financial institutions looking for a safe return on investment. UK government bonds are also known as 'Gilts'.
8 Prior to 2008, the main holders of gilts were UK pension funds and insurance companies, the Overseas Sector and other UK-based non-bank institutions. Following the introduction of QE, the APF quickly became a significant holder of gilts, rising to a peak of about 24 per cent of the total stock (over 13 per cent of GDP) by the end of 2009 (Breedon et al:2012).
9 The standard measure of the value of goods and services produced by a country during a given time period.
10 The President of the USA elected for two terms of government (1993–2001).

References

Beveridge Report (1942) *Social Insurance and Allied Services*. HMSO Cmd 6404.

Breedon, F, Chadha, J and Waters, A (2012) 'The financial market impact of UK quantitative easing' in BIS Papers no 65. *The Threat of Fiscal Dominance*. Basel. Bank for International Settlements/OECD.

Davies, W (2022) Madmen economics. *London Review of Books*, vol. 44, no. 20, 3–5.

Dörre, K, Lessenich, S and Rosa, H (2015) *Sociology, Capitalism, Critique*. London. Verso.

Epstein, G (2001) *Financialization, Rentier Interests, and Central Bank Policy*. Amherst. Department of Economics, University of Massachusetts.

Institute of Fiscal Studies (2009) *Two Parliaments of Pain*. https://ifs.org.uk/sites/default/files/2022-07/b09-public_finances.pdf (accessed 07/2022).

International Monetary Fund (2022) *Historical Public Debt database*. https://www.imf.org/external/datamapper/datasets/DEBT (accessed 10/2022).

Karwowski, E (2019) Towards (de-)financialisation: the role of the State, *Cambridge Journal of Economics*, vol. 43, no. 4, 1001–1027.

Lenin, V (1976) *State and Revolution*. Reprint. Peking. Foreign Languages Press.

McCauley, R, McGuire, P and Wooldrige, P (2021) Seven decades of international banking, *BIS Quarterly Review*, September 2021;61–75.

OECD (2021) *Government at a Glance* (2021 Edition). https://stats.oecd.org/ (accessed 09/2022).

Pierson, C (1996) *The Modern State*. London. Routledge.

Resolution Foundation & Centre for Economic Performance, LSE (2022) *Stagnation nation: Navigating a route to a fairer and more prosperous Britain*. https://economy2030.resolutionfoundation.org/reports/ (accessed 09/2022).

Smith, A (1776) *The Wealth of Nations – 2004 Reprint*. Harmondsworth. Penguin Classic.

Streek, W (2017) *Buying Time: The Delayed Crisis of Democratic Capitalism* (2nd Ed). London. Verso.

Woodward, R (1994) *The Agenda: Inside the Clinton White House*. New York. Simon & Schuster.

Wright-Mills, C (1956) *The Power Elite*. Oxford. Oxford University Press.

The process of public policy-making

What is policy?

In the French language, no distinction is made between 'policy' and 'politics', both are expressed simply as 'politique'. If 'policy' is inseparable from the 'political' (and vice versa), then formalised models of policy-making that seek to minimise the influence of political and ideological factors in the decision-making process should be treated at best with circumspection. Policy is generally understood as a course of action or *web of decisions* (Hill:1997;7) that is dynamic and therefore subject to change. But just as important, a given policy can also mean adopting a position of inaction or 'non-decision making', with the goal of maintaining the status quo. In short, policy emerges from a range of processes that may be observable involving a formal decision-making process or as the de-facto outcome of actions undertaken over a period of time which are not necessarily pre-determined or formally agreed upon.

What constitutes public policy?

The use of the term 'public policy' is generally associated with a particular course of action that reflects the intent of an elected government, as the legal authority within a given national state, in specific areas of public concern and interest. The latter would include health care, education, social protection, security and defence, and other many other areas of state activity. It therefore follows that public policy has a primacy over all other types of policies, whether these are personal or organisational. In 1999, the Labour government in the UK published a White Paper entitled *Modernising Government* that sought to set out the 'official' view of the constituents of public policy-making. This was defined 'as the process by which governments translate their political vision into programmes and actions to deliver "outcomes" – or desired changes in the real world' (Cabinet Office Strategic Policy Making Team:1999;para 2.1).

Models of public policy-making

The constitutional model

This traditional approach presents the public policy-making process as essentially a transparent process, with formal 'policy actors' having clearly specified and account-able roles at various identified 'stages' of what is termed a 'policy cycle'. In this model, three key sets of policy actors are identified (a) political parties and politicians who set out a policy programme or manifesto when standing for election to government, (b) special interest or 'advocacy' groups of all types ranging from large and powerful

DOI: 10.4324/9781003564249-4

corporate bodies through to single issue pressure groups run by volunteers, and (c) the state bureaucracy.

The process of policy-making is seen to occur in the following series of formalised stages. Politicians together with their advisors are seen to translate the political values and ideology of their political party into a series of policy proposals that are set out in an election manifesto – the legislative programme proposed by a party. These policy proposals are necessarily designed to be 'electorally friendly', and frequently without reference to long-term fiscal probity. In a general election, these policy programmes are subject to public debate and determine the basis on which the public make their choice of which party to vote for. A new government is then formed by the party whose programme is supported by the majority of the electorate or at least a majority of those who voted in a 'first-past-the-post' electoral system as is the case in the UK. Proportional representation voting systems exist in many European countries, and this often results in the formation of coalition governments. This can often make the policy formation process a fraught and complex political trade-off. Once in power, the Party of government (or several political parties within a coalition) sets out its legislative programme that in principle matches its pre-election commitments. A process of formal consultation then follows during which different special interest groups can lobby for their concerns to be incorporated into any proposed legislation. In the UK parliamentary system, the practical details of a particular policy are then drawn up by senior civil servants and set out in a published 'White Paper'. A debate in Parliament then occurs followed by a vote and the subsequent passing (or rejection) of this new legislation. The new legislation is then subject to a process of formal guidance provided by senior state officials prior to its implementation.

This simplified constitutional model raises more questions than it answers. Issues of power and influence that exist outside the formal formulation of policy process are largely absent, and the role of the state bureaucracy in the mediation or translation of policy is often played down. Special interest groups also play an important role in shaping the policy agenda of a government. The political and economic interests of powerful elite groups can often bypass the formal policy process altogether and use their influence to directly lobby politicians and state officials outside the formal consultative machinery. A special interest group such as a charity promoting the needs of a patient group can lobby government to change aspects of the proposed health policy, but they are required to participate in what is known as the lobbying system and formally declare their interests. Yet even these small single-issue pressure groups with limited resources can potentially make an impact, particularly if they cluster together with other groups to form 'issue networks'. In 2021 in the USA, some 12,137 identifiable interest groups were involved in the lobbying of the US government in Washington, DC (Holyoke:2022). In the British political system, such forms of organised lobbying are not as developed, but this does point to the importance of processes located outside the formal of representative democracy.

Weber's model of 'Rational' bureaucracy

The role played by state bureaucracies (civil service) in the policy-making process can often be an ambiguous one. State bureaucracies like to present themselves as rational and objective hierarchical structures, but the term 'bureaucracy' is also widely used in a pejorative sense, that is, bureaucracies as self-serving Kafkaesque labyrinthine structures that lack humanity. Informing these popular views (even if only implicitly and tangentially) is the classic work of Max Weber,[1] whose sociological conception of bureaucracies is universally recognised as forming the basis of the modern study of organisations and businesses.

Underpinning Weber's model of bureaucracy was his general theory of social action that presented all human action as determined by meanings and motives. Social action in pre-modern societies was seen as characterised by emotions, tradition and custom, while in modern industrialised societies, it was seen as being determined by rationality alone. Rationality for Weber was possessing a clear set of goals and a systematic assessment of the means to achieve these goals, the process of bureaucratisation being a prime example of rationality in action:

> Once fully established bureaucracy is among the structures which are hard to destroy. Bureaucracy is *the* means of transforming social action into rationally organized action. Therefore, as an instrument of rationally organised authority relations, bureaucracy was and is a power instrument of the first order for those who control the bureaucratic apparatus. Under otherwise equal conditions, rationally organized and directed action is superior to every kind of collective behaviour and also social action opposing it. Where administrations have been completely bureaucratized, the resulting system of domination is practically indestructible.
>
> *(Weber:1978;987)*

In setting out this 'ideal-type',[2] Weber identified six 'tendencies' characteristic of bureaucratic organisation, many of which still pertain in contemporary state bureaucracies: (a) A system of formalised rules and hierarchical structures. (b) The rights and duties of officials at each level are specified and remunerated accordingly. (c) Well-trained staff, appointed on the basis of their technical knowledge and expertise. (d) Promotion in the organisation based on merit with clear career pathways. (e) Impartiality of management. (f) The obedience of staff is not to an individual superior in the hierarchy, but to the 'impersonal order' that has imparted authority to this individual.

However, Weber's analysis of the spread of bureaucratic organisations should not be read as deriving solely due to their efficiency alone. He recognised that the historical development of state bureaucracies in the late nineteenth century represented the cultural constitution of the values of rationalisation, and as such constituted a new 'structure of dominance' in these societies. Yet ultimately Weber was pessimistic about what he saw as being an inexorable process, one in which the 'purely technical superiority of bureaucracy over all other forms of organization' is realised. One unintended consequence of this process was that state bureaucracies were eventually to 'become their own masters'. While the role of senior civil servants is formally that of providing the expertise for problem-solving, this role can all too easily become one of adjusting policy at a pre-implementation stage. In the twenty-first century, the question of over-bearing and politicised bureaucracies is less about the emasculation of radical political agendas, and more a concern with the growing influence of 'policy communities'. This latter development involves the increasing interaction and interchange that occurs between the top bureaucratic positions within the civil service and those in similar positions of authority within large multinational corporations. Concerns have arisen in recent years following the greater involvement of the private sector in the provision of public services.

The pragmatic model

Weber's ideal-typology held sway in the analysis of policy-making up to the middle of the twentieth century, but a more critical understanding of bureaucratic rationality emerged in the late 1950s, both in the US and British contexts. Many of these new inter-pretations of the role of state bureaucracies were normative ones, with their authors motivated by a desire to prescribe the most effective method of policy-making within public organisations (Hill:1997;98).

Herbert Simon's influential study of 'Administrative Behaviour' (1957) emphasised the essential pragmatic rationality of organisations, where decision-making was a pro-cess concerned with selecting from a range of alternative choices ranked in importance. This process of selection was about choosing an option that was able to best maximise the attainment of the core values of the organisation in question. The final decision would follow on from a comprehensive assessment of the consequences of following each of the alternative options. This pragmatic approach to policy-making required a clarity about the outcome requirements of a particular organisation, as well as the prior identification of the 'means' for achieving these ends. This was not a rejection of the idea of a rational bureaucracy, but rather an understanding of organisations as evolving 'organic' systems possessing emergent properties. This was also an acknowledgement that in practice there is little control over 'input flows' in policy-making, combined with an understanding that patterns of organisational behaviour can themselves be sources of change (Clegg:1994;62).

One of the uncertain 'input flows' identified by Simon that served to mitigate against the possibility of a completely rational policy-making process was the fact that organi-sations themselves could never be entirely homogeneous structures, as was assumed by Weber. Simon recognised that it was quite possible for the goals of individual deci-sion-makers to differ from that of the organisation as a whole. This was an acknowl-edgement of the difficulties associated with any prior specification of ends and the identification of means to achieve these ends. It was on this basis that Simon conceded that only a limited degree of 'bounded rationality' was possible within state bureaucra-cies. This was also a reflection of the fact (but missing in Simon's own model) that the goals and values of state bureaucratic organisations are in themselves policies and so are themselves continually subject to dispute and change (Hill:2004;146).

The incremental model

Simon's pragmatic model was soon to be challenged by those who argued that in prac-tice policy-making decisions were made incrementally. That is, organisational decision-making proceeded on the basis of limiting the number of policy alternatives to be considered to those only marginally different from existing policies (rather than the full range of alternatives envisaged in Simon's model). This position known as the Incrementalist model (also known more colloquially as the 'muddling through' model), followed the work of Braybrooke and Lindblom (1963) and their understanding of the limited problem-solving capacities of bureaucratic organisations. These limitations included inadequate access to appropriate feedback data and information; failure to develop satisfactory evaluation and assessment methods; and the sheer multiplicity of contexts and variables within which an organisation operates.

The primary motivation underpinning Braybrooke and Lindblom's work was not only to evaluate processes of policy-making, but also to develop a prescriptive model for organisational decision-making. The authors asserted that serious mistakes could be avoided if only small changes were made in policy development at any one time. The assertion being that 'muddling-through' best suited the pluralistic process (the standard uncritical model of American politics in the 1950s and 1960s) of bargaining and negotiation between the different interest groups within the US political system. However, the deductive power of this model was limited by the difficulties it faced in determining what actually constituted an 'increment', the size of changes that are and could be made within a given policy. The model also assumed that decision-making processes were stable over time. In practice, what are known as 'shift-points' or a fundamental rethinking about the course of policy development occur, and these often defy incrementalist equations (Lane:2000;76).

'Public Choice' model

This particular model of public policy-making has its origins in neoliberal thought, although in practice it represents a slight shift away from the classic models of rational choice that are drawn upon as a critique of state welfare state provision.[3] Public choice theory recognises the state as a 'rational actor' pursuing a 'logic of interest' and on this basis seeks to explain the motivations and interests that lie behind the policy decision-making behaviour of politicians and other state actors. Nordhaus (1975) and Mueller (1979, 1989) have argued that incumbent governments will seek to stimulate the economy before an General Election by increasing spending on programmes that appeal most to the electorate in order to get re-elected. They will then deflate the economy after the election by raising taxes or reducing public deficits by some other means in order to fulfil their electoral promises. Although public choice models do not lack political plausibility and have undoubtedly been very influential they often lack an empirical basis for their conclusions. The models also tend to over-emphasise the supply side in public policy-making. That is, they focus on what are seen to be excessive budget allocations for the supply of public services, and not on the demands of the voters and the extent to which more socially deprived groups benefit through redistributive programmes, transferring payments from high- to low-income groups (Lane:2000;90). A further criticism is that the model assumes the existence of a fixed set of preferences for political actors to choose from, it then finds it difficult to account for why public institutions do change over time (Schmidt:2006;103).

The 'Garbage Can' model

By the 1980s, attempts to assess decision-making as a rational or linear incremental set of processes, as well as to construct prescriptive or normative models of the most effective forms of bureaucratic action, were being challenged by the self-styled 'Garbage Can' model (Olsen:1983). Olsen's approach presented itself as more realistic representation of the constraints to rationalism within public organisations (as indeed do all the other models that were discussed above) and emphasised the apparent irrational and chaotic reality of decision-making behaviour. Olsen identified a range of less than rational ideal-typological features of organisational policy-making that included uncertain knowledge about outcomes, and decision-making rules that were largely symbolic. The conclusion subsequently drawn by March and Olsen (1986) was that the complexity of organisational policy-making was unlikely ever to be captured by a single model. It was on the basis of this critical standpoint that these same authors went on to re-orientate their analysis towards the emergence of 'in-and-of-themselves' organisational structures (what they termed institutional 'logics'), which were seen to guide the decision-making process (March & Olsen:1989;160). This approach morphed into what subsequently became known as 'Institutional theory', also known as 'historical institutionalism', or sometimes to just plain 'institutionalism'.

Institutional theory and the path-dependency of public policy

The re-orientation within policy studies towards a more explicit institutionalist approach to the understanding of the development public policy began in the 1990s. This was in response to the growing criticism of the de-contextualised and narrow scope of the existing models that were described above. As ideal-type policy-making models consistently failed account for the ambiguity (and 'garbage') that frequently accompanied the decision-making processes, so Institutional theory began to exert a strong influence in the study of complex organisations such as health care systems. The key assumption of this emergent field of analysis is the specificity of historically constructed institutional constraints that ultimately serve to influence (wittingly or not) the behaviour of policy actors in the decision-making process. Institutionalism offered the possibility of explaining why there is often resistance to policy change, what sustains a policy status quo, and the ways in which in-built barriers to institutional change are maintained over time.

Institutional theory presents the politics of the national state ('the polity'), as the 'primary locus for action, yet understands political activities, whether carried by politicians or by social groups, as conditioned by institutional configurations of governments and party political systems' (Skocpol:1992;41). Its essential insight is that formal rules and structures can merge with informal, non-codified rules and practices within state institutions (Thornton & Ocasio 2008). This position is in complete contrast to the assumptions of public choice theory that each state actor in the policy process (politicians, interest groups, bureaucrats, etc.) has the ability to make strategic, calculated actions in pursuance of their own self, group or class interest. Institutionalism asserts that policy-making activities are not only historically bounded and constrained, but that institutional rules systematically privilege particular policy actors. As summed up by W. Richard Scott, this is 'the way we (the institution) do things' (Scott:2001;57). It is, therefore, a structured approach that recognises the autonomy of key political actors, while acknowledging the influence of previously enacted policies on the decision-making process engaged in by these same actors.

Institutionalism as a field of study seeks to delineate: 'The origins and development of institutional structures and processes over time. It tends to focus on sequences in development, timing of events, and phases of political change. It emphasizes not just the asymmetries of power related to the operation and development of institutions but also the path-dependencies and unintended consequences that result from such historical development' (Schmidt:2006;105).

A key concept arising from Institutional theory is known as 'path-dependency' which refers to the dynamics of a self-reinforcing or positive feedback processes in public policy-making. This concept points to the ways in which policy options in the present are constrained by institutional structures that were constructed in the past. Once a path of activity is chosen, it is difficult to change direction as institutional decision-making processes become reinforced over time. For Mahoney (2000), the process of path-dependency has deterministic properties. The identification of path-dependence within the policy-making process of any given state institution involves tracing a given policy outcome back to a particular historical chain of events, while also showing how these events are themselves contingent occurrences that cannot be explained only on the basis of prior historical conditions (Mahoney:2000;507–508). By definition, path-dependency is difficult to alter so there are strong incentives to continue in a particular policy direction. In order to avoid this outcome it becomes important for organisations to build in self-evaluation structures that enable policy adaptation in the changing context in which a particular institution operates.

Paul Pierson (2000) has argued that institutional path-dependency as a historical process has three distinct phases. Firstly, 'small' events early on in a pathway ('incrementalism') can subsequently have disproportionately large effects in shaping the long-term trajectory of institutional policy development. Secondly, during the early stages of a sequence, a 'critical juncture' may occur where the policy pathway becomes restrictive in some way. Thirdly, as a policy pathway is followed, '... previously viable options may be foreclosed' as self-reinforcing feedback mechanisms encourage the move along one particular policy direction (Pierson:2000;81). This notion of phases to path-dependency embraces a particular casual logic that emphasises the lasting impact of unanticipated exogenous shocks on the adoption of a particular institutional policy courses.[4] This combination of critical conjunctures and path-dependence has been termed the 'dual model' of institutional development (Capoccia & Kelemen:2007;341), yet there are many analysts who would describe this approach as conceptually inconsistent.

It is always methodologically challenging to attempt to combine two distinct mechanisms in one analytical framework, yet this is what Kathleen Thelen and her collaborators have attempted to achieve over the course of the last two decades.[5] Thelen's position is that over time relatively small changes can have a cumulative effect on the direction of travel of institutional policy-making while at the same time, she also emphasises the role of a whole typology of policy actors known as 'change agents'. Together these elements constitute 'both continuity and structured change' within institutions (Thelen:1999;384). 'Change agents' are identified as being of four possible ideal-types: (a) 'insurrectionaries', (b) 'symbionts', (c) 'subversives', and (d) 'opportunists', with each linked to a distinctive mode of policy change. The influence of these change agents is in turn dependent on whether a given state institution affords these political actors considerable or few opportunities for exercising discretion in interpreting or enforcing the policy status quo (Mahoney & Thelen:2010).

This combined approach is seen to enable the development of 'nuanced descriptions and analyses of incremental change at various institutional levels (including policy and regulatory regimes), in a wide variety of contexts' (Van der Heijden & Kuhlmann:2016;538). Yet while the latter are broadly supportive of the approach of Thelen and her collaborators, they are also concerned with just how successfully it has been when applied within empirical policy research given the ambiguities of the notion of the 'change agent'. In their own research that assessed the application of Thelan's model, these authors found that there was 'a gap between theoretical expectations and empirical findings ... (resulting from the application) of a narrow set of explanatory characteristics ... (so that) it was unlikely that the theory is capable of fully explaining observed instances of incremental change' (Van der Heijden & Kuhlmann:2016;546). In short, this critique points to the limitations that inevitably follow the uncritical application of ideal-types in policy studies.

Power analysis in public policy research

An important criticism levelled at Institutional theory is that there is often an absence of any explicit analysis of power in accounts of policy development. This critique relates to the structuring of policy choices as well as accounting for policy change, beyond any particular role for 'change agents' in public institutions. As Topp et al have argued, integrating a theoretical understanding of power relations within health policy research is a necessity for the following three reasons: 'First, it provides a deeper, more nuanced understanding of the mechanisms and structures that lead to social inequities and health disparities. Second, it reveals historical patterns entrenched in health and social systems, allowing contemporary policy concerns to be seen in a wider context and lessons to be drawn from these trends. Third, analysing power can contribute to the (re)design or reform of health systems to redress imbalances and progress towards improved health outcomes' (Topp et al:2021;2). One possible explanation for the marginalisation of power analysis in public policy studies is that 'power' itself is very much a contested construct. There is a strong argument in favour of 'examining the relative power of those who directly benefit from any particular policy, those who are disadvantaged by it as direct targets, and those third parties for whom there will be indirect positive or negative effects. Policy typologies do no more than help to draw our attention to the identities of these parties' (Hill & Hupe:2014;80).

Lowi's (1964, 1972) typology of power was developed more than half a century ago, but it still continues to be widely cited as a foundational approach within political science. Theodore Lowi focused on what can best be described as the 'macro' level of governmental and institutional structures of governance and authority, rather than the 'micro' level, as represented by the discretionary power that may be exercised by the chief executive of a health care provider trust for example. Theodore Lowi's distinct contribution was in recognising that 'for every type of policy there is likely to be a distinctive type of political relationship' (1964;688). It was on this basis that he framed public policy as essentially a process of top-down coercion that required organisations to adopt particular courses of action (Lowi:1964;689). Lowi went onto develop four policy option types, these are set out below and include illustrative examples drawn from contemporary health policy (but not in relation to his fourth type for the reasons also set out below).

(a) *Regulatory*: Regulations are the restrictions imposed upon the activities of both institutions and individual citizens and include forms of guidance, all normally backed up by force of sanctions. Regulatory policies prescribe negative sanctions for not adjusting to an authorised norm. In health policy this might relate to the restrictions and controls placed on health care institutions such as setting quality standards for the treatment and care of patients and subject to regular inspection; licensing arrangements and approval of medications; patient safety standards; qualifications and training requirements for health care staff; etc.

(b) *Distributive:* Policies predicated on the basis of the principle that particular services such as health care, education, social protection and security are 'public goods' which benefit all citizens. These services are best provided by the state in order that all citizens may have access whatever their income or wealth. Distributive health policies are most apparent in those countries that have tax-funded universal health service provision and equity of access.

(c) *Redistributive:* This type of policy goes further than distributive policies in that they expressly seek to re-balance the distribution of income, wealth and power in a given society. In health care terms, redistributive policies could include prioritising the narrowing of social inequalities in health outcome. This could be at the level of the individual need or it could mean a redistribution of resources to those regions with the highest level of demand.

Lowi's focus on policy implementation as differentially applied forms of coercive power, reflected his recognition that a substantive asymmetrical relationship existed between the authority and power of the state and the ordinary citizens in any given country. This was a position that was at odds with the dominant pluralistic view of the state-citizen relationship that held sway within US politics in the 1960s when Lowi was writing. This political ideology of pluralism was one that reflected Max Weber's classic statement, that '(I)n general, we understand by power the chance of a man or a number of men to realize their own will in a communal action even against the resistance of others who are participating in the action' (Weber:1978;926). Although Lowi explicitly identifies policy as the exercise of power, an important element of his model was the relative 'likelihood' of coercion being exerted in the implementation of any given public policy. Here Lowi was embracing the view that power could be exercised without there being any observable coercion or conflict, and that individual or institutional changes could be induced through a range of means not just formal sanctions. In part this reflected the influence of Robert Dahl and his much quoted statement that; '*A* has power over *B* to the extent that he can get *B* to do something that *B* would not otherwise do' (Dahl:1957). At the core of Lowi's typology is a conceptualisation of power as domination, manifested in successful acts of policy implementation. Yet Lowi's work has subsequently been critiqued on the basis that it was too focused on the relational elements of the exercise of power in policy-making and down-playing the structural factors in play.

The work of Steven Lukes (2004) sought to extend Lowi's typology of power in relation to the formulating of public policy options. For Lukes, power is as much a potentiality as an actuality, in that it does not need to be observed in order to exist. Measuring 'power resources' such as wealth, status and political influence can provide evidence of how power is distributed within a given society, but power is primarily, '... a *capacity* and not the exercise or the vehicle of that capacity' (2004;70). In his influential study Lukes identified three potential 'dimensions' of power, each of which is discussed in detail below.

The *One-dimensional* view of power is essentially the 'regulatory' conceptualisation identified in Lowi's typology. It is termed one-dimensional because it focuses exclusively on observable behaviour, whereby one group prevails over another in decision-making situations. This reflects a Weberian concern with agential social action to the exclusion of the role of institutional structures in decision-making processes. While this view of power offers a relatively straightforward pathway for policy studies because of its focus on the observable decision-making of key political agents, for Lukes it is essentially blind to the ways in which a policy agenda is controlled (1974:58).

The *Two-dimensional* view of power was established on the basis of Lukes' critique of the work of Bachrach and Baratz (1970). The latter had asserted that those who hold power within the public policy-making process were those with the authority to be able to choose between decision-making or non-decision-making. Non-decision-making is exercised when particular courses of action are actively prevented from being placed on a policy agenda. Lukes's (1974) critique is that while the two-dimensional view moves beyond an exclusive focus on formal decision-making behaviour, it continues to place too much emphasis on the actions of individuals within the decision-making system. He argued that attention should also be given to the ways in which these actions themselves reflect the socially structured and culturally patterned behaviour of those holding authority (1974;22). Both the one- and the two-dimensional views presuppose that power is only exercised in situations of actual conflict between different interest groups, yet this often fails to acknowledge that, 'the most effective and insidious use of power is to prevent such conflict from arising in the first place' (1974:23). Lukes argued that it was a mistake to assume that non-decision-making power, '... only exists where there are grievances which are denied entry into the political process in the form of issues' (1974;24).

Lukes' *Third dimension* applies when power is exercised to manipulate and shape the wants, needs, and norms of a given population. This is achieved through the hegemony (or leadership) of a dominant social group in the social hierarchy. The latter exercise their power through their control over ideological structures such as the education system, the media, and various other socialisation processes. This is a view of power that focuses not only on overt or covert observable conflict, but also the potential for 'latent conflict' between 'subjective and real interests' arising from the decision or policymaking process (Lukes:2004;29).[6]

The relationship between the policy-making and policy implementation

The notion of policy 'implementation' generally refers to the execution of an outcome, whether or not that outcome is consistent with the original intentions of the policymakers (Lane:2000;98). In the past, the public policy literature tended to blur any distinction between the formulation of a set of policy objectives and the process of implementation, both being conceived as linked stages of a 'policy cycle'. This long-held assumption was only reluctantly let go, when empirical evidence was able to demonstrate there was frequently a distinct lack of correspondence between formal policy objectives and actual policy outcomes. This was the de facto recognition of the so-called 'Implementation deficit'. The empirical recognition of a 'deficit' reflected the fact that the relationship between the formation of policy and its implementation, as well as the outcomes of that policy was a far more complex one than that represented in rationalistic assumptions concerning the policy process as a series of linear stages. The recognition of an implementation deficit led onto the development of alternative approaches manifest in the so-called 'top-down' and 'bottom-up' models.

The 'top-down' model focuses attention on the relations of authority in any given large-scale public institution seen as the primary mechanism for successful implementation of any policy. The model also sought to identify the limits to control inherent in these complex public institutions, for example the National Health Service (NHS), so that they could be more effectively managed. The 'top-down' model presumes that policy-making is a 'one-shot' process that involves a clearly defined entity, 'the policy', in its entirety. But as Hill (2004;182) has noted, it is difficult to determine where the formal policy-making process ends and implementation of that policy begins, and he cites the following reasons for this view: (a) Conflicts of interest cannot be resolved at the policy-making stage. (b) Key decisions can only be made when all the facts are available to policy implementers. (c) Certain groups of agents charged with the process of policy implementation (professional managers, for example) are better equipped to make key decisions than others. (d) Policy-makers can only make educated guesses about the actual impact of new policies. (e) The day-to-day task of implementation inevitably involves negotiation and compromise with conflicting sets of interests on-going throughout the life of a policy. (f) Finally, it may be considered politically inexpedient for central government to intervene directly to resolve the local conflicts arising out the implementation of a national policy.

The claim made for 'bottom-up' models is that of analytical realism. In examining the translation of policy objectives into organisational practice, this model 'focuses attention on the structures of discretion and autonomy afforded to local managers and to the relevant professionals at the so-called 'street-level' of policy implementation' (Hill & Hupe:2014;57). Here the concern is focused on the 'concrete behaviour' of those lower down the institutional hierarchy charged with carrying out policy. At this 'street level', actors are faced with making choices between new and existing policy programmes that may conflict or interact with one another. This requires what Elmore (1979) has described in his influential paper as a 'backward mapping' approach to implementation.

Over time, both these models have been subject to critical analysis on the basis that they share the same basic standpoint, that policy formation and policy implementation were separate elements of a policy cycle. Yet in the 'world of implementation ... there is not always a straight line going from identified problem to realized solution' (Hill & Hupe:2014;165). So rather than focusing on why policy implementation 'deficits' occur, an alternative approach was to develop an understanding of implementation as a dynamic *process* (rather than as a linear process), capable of both adding to or subtracting from policy goals. It was on this basis that Winter (2006;159) argued that research studies should redirect their focus towards policy outcomes rather than the achievement of identified formal policy goals. This consideration led onto a new concern with relationships of governance in the development of public policy. Governance in relation to health policy is the focus of the next chapter.

Notes

1 Max Weber (1864–1920) was a German social theorist who arguably has been one of the most influential figures in the development of sociological theory and political philosophy in the twentieth century.
2 'Ideal-types' are methodological tools utilised for analytical purposes and represent the attempt to capture social reality through the process of classification and systemisation. In short they are simplified schemas of the workings of the social world.
3 Discussed in detail in Chapter 1.
4 The COVID-19 pandemic can be seen as an example of such a critical juncture, which then shifted the dial, so to speak, away from decentralised processes of health resource management back to a command-and-control model of system governance – see also Chapter 3 on this point.
5 Mahoney and Thelen's *Explaining Institutional Change* (2010) has been cited over 3,000 times according to Google Scholar (as of December 2022).
6 See Chapter 10 for an application of Lukes's model in relation to the influence of the pharmaceutical industry within health policymaking.

References

Bachrach, P and Baratz, M (1970) *Power and Poverty: Theory and Practice*. New York. Oxford University Press.
Braybrooke, D and Lindblom, C (1963) *A Strategy of Decision*. New York. Free Press.
Cabinet Office Strategic Policy Making Team (1999) *Professional Policy Making for the Twenty-First Century*. https://intouk.files.wordpress.com
Capoccia, G and Kelemen, D (2007) The study of critical conjunctures: Theory, narrative. *World Politics*, vol. 59, no. 3, 341–369.
Clegg, S (1994) 'Max Weber and the contemporary sociology of organisations' in Ray, L and Reed, M (eds) *Organizing Modernity: New Weberian Perspectives on Work, Organization and Society*. London. Routledge, pp 46–80.
Dahl, RA (1957) *The Concept of Power*. New York. Bobbs-Merrill.
Elmore, R (1979) Backward mapping: implementation research and policy decision, *Political Science Quarterly*, vol. 94, no. 4, 601–616.
Hill, M (1997) *The Policy Process in the Modern State* (3rd Ed). London. Prentice-Hall.
Hill, M (2004) *The Public Policy Process* (4th Ed). Harlow. Pearson Longman.
Hill, M and Hupe, P (2014) *Implementing Public Policy* (3rd Ed). London. Sage.
Holyoke, T (2022) *Our lobbyists don't always advocate for what we want them to* (January 21, 2022). https://blogs.lse.ac.uk.
Lane, JE (2000) *The Public Sector: Concepts, Models and Approaches* (3rd Ed). London. Sage.
Lowi, T (1964) American Business, public policy, case studies, and political theory, *World Politics*, vol. 16, 677–715.
Lowi, T (1972) Four systems of policy, politics and choice, *Public Administration Review*, vol. 32, 298–310.
Lukes, S (1974) *Power: A Radical View*. Basingstoke. Macmillan.
Lukes, S (2004) *Power: A Radical View* (2nd Ed). London. Palgrave.
Mahoney, J (2000) Path dependence in historical sociology. *Theory and Society*, vol. 29, 507–548.
Mahoney, J and Thelen, K (2010) 'A theory of gradual institutional change' in Mahoney, J and Thelen, K (eds) *Explaining Institutional Change: Ambiguity, Agency, and Power*. Cambridge. Cambridge University Press, pp. 1–37
March, J and Olsen, J (1986) 'Garbage can models of decision-making in organizations' in March, J and Weissinger-Baylon, R (eds) *Ambiguity and Command: Organizational Perspectives on Military Decision Making*. Marshfield, MA: Pitman, pp. 11–35.
March, J and Olsen, J (1989) *Rediscovering Institutions: The Organizational Basis of Politics*. New York. Free Press.
Mueller, D (1979) *Public Choice*. Cambridge. Cambridge University Press.
Mueller, D (1989) *Public Choice II*. Cambridge. Cambridge University Press.
Nordhaus, W (1975) The political business cycle, *Review of Economic Studies*, vol. 42, 169–190.

Olsen, J (1983) *Organised Democracy*. Oslo. Universitetsforlaget.

Pierson, P (2000) Not just what, but when: timing and sequence in political processes, *Studies in American Political Development*, vol. 14, 72–92.

Schmidt, V (2006) 'Institutionalism' in Hay, C. Lister, M and Marsh, D (eds) *The State: Theories and Issues*. Basingstoke. Palgrave Macmillan, pp 98–117.

Scott, W (2001) *Institutions and Organisations* (2nd Ed). London. Sage.

Simon, HA (1957) *Administrative Behaviour* (2nd Ed). New York. Macmillan.

Skocpol, T (1992) *Protecting Soldiers and Mothers*. Cambridge, MA. Harvard University Press.

Thelen, K (1999) Historical institutionalism in comparative politics, *Annual Review of Political Science*, vol. 2, 369–404.

Thornton, P and Ocasio, W (2008) 'Institutional order' in Greenwood, R, Salin-Andersson, O and Suddaby, R (eds) *The Sage Handbook of Organizational Institutionalism*. London: Sage, pp 99–129.

Topp, S, Schaaf, M, Sriram, V, et al (2021) Power analysis in health policy and systems research: a guide to research conceptualisation, *BMJ Global Health*, vol. 6, e007268.

Van der Heijden, J and Kuhlmann, J (2016) Studying incremental institutional change: a systematic and critical meta review of the literature 2005–2015, *Policy Studies Journal*, vol. 45, no. 3, 535–554.

Weber, M (1978) *Economy and Society (2 Volumes)*. Berkeley. University of California Press.

Winter, S (2006) 'Implementation' in Peters, B and Pierre, J (eds) *Handbook of Public Policy*. London. Sage, pp 151–166.

CHAPTER 3

The governance of health care systems

Conceiving governance in the policy process

At its core, the notion of 'governance' is essentially a heuristic, a shorthand that is utilised in order to denote the complex and dynamic sets of relational processes that occur within institutions and organisations. Yet the term has an inherent 'slipperiness' that makes it difficult to settle on any one definitive conceptualisation able to fit all analytical contexts. This slipperiness is reflected in the fact that a further set of constructs are frequently deployed in order to provide a definition of sorts, these include 'relationships', 'authority', 'steering', 'accountability', 'transparency', 'regulation', and 'constraint'. Yet these attempts at simplifying the meaning of 'governance' often result in the opposite effect, obfuscation. Nevertheless, in recent decades, governance as a concept has appeared with increasing frequency in the public and health policy literature, and in this role, it is frequently required to do a lot of analytical heavy lifting.

What the notion of governance is decidedly *not* is a systematic theory of power and authority, and when it is utilised in analysis it should at best be regarded as an 'umbrella term' used to represent what has been termed 'government-in-action' (Hill & Hupe:2014;117). In the same vein, it can also be used to convey, 'a capacity for getting things done which is not captured in any simple way by the power of government to command' (Davies et al:2005;82).

One application of the term to be found within public policy analysis is the attempt to construct a framework or template for constructing 'effective' institutional practices. Such templates are often used as the basis for the reform of institutional structures seen as characterised by organisational corruption, systemic failure to learn from errors, lack of public accountability in decision-making, and the inefficient use of public resources. The shorthand phrase that is frequently drawn upon in describing this state of affairs is 'bad governance'. Templates for 'good governance' generally focus attention on how best to vertically remodel organisational decision-making structures so that they include appropriate internal controls, long-term strategic development, and stakeholder representation (Greer et al:2016;11).

The increasing prominence of the term 'governance' can also be explained in part, by its use in situating the changes that are perceived to have occurred in the traditional social and structural relationships pertaining between individual citizens and the state. These social and organisational processes are generally seen as emergent from the late 1980s onwards, and collectively conceived as a process of 'post-modernity'.[1] The latter construct being used to depict a world in which traditional social and cultural hierarchies are seen as having been eroded. A world where the vertical, command-and-control decision-making role of the state is displaced and in its stead have emerged

DOI: 10.4324/9781003564249-5

horizontal, self-organised 'communication networks', facilitated by the new digitalised social media. In practice, this was a distorted and essentially prescriptive analysis that never came close to being fulfilled. The notion of a 'networked' democracy was essentially a self-constructed myth that overplayed the extent to which these traditional hierarchies of power and authority had actually been undermined (Davies:2022;2). While the once all-conquering conception of postmodernity has largely evaporated from social and cultural analysis, the associated concept of governance continues to be drawn upon in the analysis of the exercise of authority.

Embracing governance as a dynamic and non-linear conceptualisation of the infrastructure of decision-making within institutions does have the benefit of enabling policy analyses to move beyond 'stagist' and overly formalised models of the policy process. The notion of governance is able to incorporate the complexities associated with the exercise of power and authority as it exists between a wide range of policy actors, both within and outside the institutions of government. Hill and Hupe (2014) have attempted to capture this dynamic in their *multi-governance* framework, designed for the analysis of 'government-in-action'. The connective elements of this framework include a number of distinct 'levels' which are described below (Hill & Hupe:2014;128–130):

(i) *Actors:* Seen to be those officials or organisations to whom a 'task has been mandated'.
(ii) *Administrative layers:* Referring to the 'locations' of action, which are not necessarily predicated on a specific or formal role of any given administrative or political layer of the state.
(iii) *Action levels*: Consisting of three arenas of decision-making. The first of these is termed *constitutive* where decisions about decision rules are made. The second is termed *directional* and concerns the path that 'collectively desired outcomes' of a particular policy should take, while the third is termed *operational* and refers to 'the actual managing' or realisation of a particular policy.
(iv) *Action situations:* This level draws attention to the specific form that each of the three 'action levels' described above take. This is seen to be dependent on the particular 'locus' or scale of the policy process. So 'action situations' can include the *individual* or 'street level' of interaction between state officials; the *organisational* level, for example involving the diverse management as well as health professional decision-making committees that compose a hospital trust for example; and at the *system* level, where decision-making processes take place.
(v) *Political-administrative craftsmanship:* This level refers to the 'quality of human agency', or simply put, can actor 'A' carry out a task more effectively than actor 'B'?

Hill and Hope's (2014) multi-level governance framework, as applied to the process of developing and implementing health care policy would include a particularly wide cast of actors, both inter- and intra-organisational all engaged in a complex, but connected set of activities. Yet as Newman (2001) has pointed out, such overlapping modes of decision-making governance applied to complex organisation's such as the National Health Service (NHS) are as likely to produce a whole range of tensions as much as solutions and these ultimately have to be resolved on the ground by health practitioners themselves.

The 'New Public Management'

One of the defining features of the process of 'modernisation'[2] associated with the reform of state-funded health and welfare services in the late 1980s was a re-orientation towards organisational 'performance' and measurable system 'outcomes'. This 'revolution' was to be led by a new managerial cadre charged with instigating a 'business-like' approach to the delivery of public services. This development in essence is what became widely known as the New Public Management (NPM). The NPM was intended to gradually replace the bureaucratic layer of 'administrators' that had been in existence prior to the establishment of the NHS and who were responsible for executing top-down instructions in the day-to-day running of local health care organisations. The introduction of a new results-driven calculative managerial cadre represented 'a shift in discretionary power linked to institutional decision-making that previously has been associated with "professional calculus" but was now to be attached to managerial prerogatives' (Clarke:1998;176). New frameworks of governance were introduced that functioned to prioritise the performance requirements of the health system over all other concerns, including that of the medical profession.

NPM-style organisational reforms gradually became institutionalised within state-funded health and welfare sectors in the UK and across equivalent state service sectors in Europe from the late 1980s onwards (Hood & Scott:2000). Yet this was an uneven process, frequently resisted by service professionals, but ultimately successful given the determination of governments in high-income countries to restructure their state health and welfare services. Dunleavy et al (2006) identified three characteristic components of this process within the organisation of state services:

(a) *Incentivisation*: Manifest in the introduction of systems of performance-related pay as well as mandate contracts for managers that replaced the flat state salaries of career civil servants. This 'business-like' approach was also reflected in changes to an organisational cultural that had been focused around meeting the service needs of patients and clients, the esoteric notion of a 'service ethic', and redirecting the commitment of staff towards the needs of goals of the organisation itself.

(b) *Competition*: This market principle as the basis for bringing to an end the situation where public organisations were both the funders and providers of services. The argument was that promoting competition through a process of outsourcing service provision to external actors, be they in the public or private sector, would improve efficiency and reduce costs. This goal was to be achieved through the construction of quasi-markets, where the funding of service providers became dependent on their performance and delivery, with 'money following choice'.

(c) *Disaggregation*: This process is characterised by the 'contracting-out' of public services to profit and non-profit agencies alike. This in turn required public organisations to take on the role of 'commissioners' rather than deliverer's of services. This process has been conceptualised as the 'agentification' of those health and welfare service institutions that formally were both funders and providers of services.

Additional to Dunleavy et al's (2006) three identified characteristics of the NPM, two further characteristics can also be added:

(d) *Measurable outputs*: Developing indices of organisational performance as proxy measures for quality of care, efficiency, and effectiveness of interventions.
(e) *Organisation of work*: The emergence of new forms of authority and control within public service institutions leading onto a re-organisation of the division of labour as between specialist and non-specialist occupations. Hierarchical relationships within these organisations were gradually re-structured, reflected in changes to occupational roles, responsibilities, and established working practices.

The organisational forms that were adopted in the NPM reforms varied markedly across European Welfare states; '(S)tate modernizers, like the Nordic countries, emphasizing the contribution of reforms to a strong state and active citizenship, while marketising governments like the UK referring to a retreat of the state, selling off all non-essential State tasks' (Pollitt et al:2007;3). One position that most critical commentators can agree upon is that these reforms introduced the calculative practices of 'managerialism' into the provision and governance of public services for the first time. Arguably, this development was ultimately to lead to a reframing of the role of the state in the universal provision of public services (Clarke:2004;125). A further area of broad agreement that can also be found in the literature is that the introduction of the NPM represented a 'critical juncture' in the 'path-dependency' of public service organisations.[3] It represented the imposition from outside of a completely new doctrine of public service organisational decision-making that arguably gave precedence to system performance over all other demands.

A case study in regulation and governance: the medical profession
Doctors have always played a pivotal role in modern health care systems, reflecting their knowledge, training, expertise, and social status as a professional occupational group. The institutional history of this profession is a fascinating example of how health care governance systems have changed over time in response to emergent social and economic realities.

Health care systems require a wide range of occupational groups in order to manage, treat and care for patients A list of current health occupations would include, but not be limited to, doctors, nurses, dentists, pharmacists, midwives, occupational therapists, speech therapists, physiotherapists, psychotherapists, sonographers, radiographers, paramedics, dieticians, and opticians. The International Labour Office Standard Classification of Occupations (ISCO-08) includes all the occupations listed above, which are recognised as meeting 'Skill Level 4', the ILO requirement for classification as a 'profession'. These requirements include: '(T)he performance of tasks that require complex problem-solving, decision-making and creativity based on an extensive body of theoretical and factual knowledge in a specialized field. The skills and knowledge required for competent performance at this skill level are usually obtained as the result of study at a higher educational institution for a period of 3–6 years leading to the award of a degree or higher qualification' (ILO:2012;13).

This ISCO-8 classification reflects a lineage of occupational taxonomies that can be traced back to the 1950s. These classificatory systems are constructed on the basis of prescriptive lists of generalised social attributes or 'traits' traditionally associated with professional work. But these 'traits' often uncritically reflect the ways in which occupational groups themselves choose to present their roles as 'professional', rather than the realities of everyday work practices (Saks:2012;3). By the 1970s, a sociological approach had emerged to challenge this classificatory approach. This new understanding largely derived from the work of Max Weber, whose dense and rich social analysis of the functioning of the capitalist market economy at the turn of twentieth centuries remains influential to this day.[4] Weber's key assumption was that societies were constituted as individuals pursued their own interests, this eventually resulted in the formation of a range of more or less collectively conscious social groups. In furthering their common interests, these groups were seen as having engaged in self-serving 'social closure' strategies designed to exclude competing groups, so establishing for themselves social and economic privileges, status, and power. Occupational professions such as the Law, Medicine, Architecture and Accountancy were seen to be the archetypal examples of occupational groups that were able to develop and maintain their occupational boundaries in a marketplace of skills, so establishing their social dominance.

Elliott Friedson's (1970) analysis of the medical profession was an early example of Weber's model applied to health systems. This influential study argued that the power of doctors within modern societies derived less from any social consensus concerning the value of the profession's expertise and knowledge, and more on the profession's ability to pursue a 'social closure' strategy. This strategy was realised through the power of the profession to control not only its own work activities, but also to exercise its authority over the activities of other health care occupations such as nurses. This authority is generally known as 'clinical autonomy'. In Britain, the privileged status of the profession was firmly instituted with the establishment of the so-called historical 'social contract' embodied in the Medical Act of 1858, otherwise known as *An Act to Regulate the Qualifications of Practitioners in Medicine and Surgery*. The 'contract' between the emergent medical profession and the state was solidified in the new the creation of legal framework that enforced the de facto closed entry and occupational boundaries of the profession. The quid pro quo was that the medical profession committed itself to regulating the practice of its members via the newly created General Medical Council (GMC), so that it met its social obligation to provide competent and ethically altruistic treatment for patients (or at least to those privileged few who could afford their services in the late nineteenth century). This legislation firmly established the medical profession's position of dominance in an emerging modern system of health care and 'was both instrumentally and symbolically the sign that state power now stood behind those who controlled the GMC' (Moran:2004;29). Similar social contracts were established in North America and Western Europe in the same historical period. In Britain, oversight of the activities of individual doctors was to come via a so-called 'trinity' of regulatory instruments that included the criminal law, civil liability, but above all by its self-regulatory body, the GMC. This 'trinity' was established on the premise of the existence of competent, ethical, and autonomous professionals (McDonald:2012;106).

When following the end of the Second World War, the Labour government moved to establish a national health care system constructed on the basis of universal and free provision based only on health need, it was initially opposed by the profession's representative body, the British Medical Association (BMA). This was on the basis that a universal system would extend state regulatory control over the activities and autonomy of the profession and lead to a loss of lucrative private practice opportunities; this turned out to be a misplaced fear. The newly established NHS depended entirely upon the clinical knowledge, experience and skills of doctors, and from this position of strength, the BMA was able to negotiate favourable terms for the participation of General Practitioners and hospital Consultants. Within the new NHS, senior doctors were given effective control over the day-to-day allocation of resources and staff, while the role of the state was confined to deciding the level of overall state funding. However, as the scope of the financial commitment to health care expanded in the 1970s and 1980s to meet ever-increasing demands, so the dominance of this self-regulated profession came to be seen as a barrier to improving the efficiency of the organisation.

In the late nineteenth and early twentieth centuries, Germany had followed a broadly similar pattern of professionalisation and self-regulation, but this was marked by a much closer relationship of governance pertaining between the profession and the newly centralised German state than was the case in Britain. As Michael Moran explains: 'The historical British strategy might be summed up as the creation of a private governing world enclosed from the wider world of the state and the market: the German strategy involved the use of powerful self-governing institutions to intervene in that wider world' (Moran:1999;110). Drawing on a historical institutionalist perspective,[5] Moran argues that the early close working relationship between the state and profession in Germany led onto the development of a much more complex and nuanced system of regulation and governance later in the twentieth century. This was the period that followed the defeat of Nazism and the end of the Second World War, which saw a reemergence of democracy, the establishment of a universal health care system, and the creation of what became known as the 'corporatist state'.[6]

The organisational restructuring linked to the introduction of the NPM saw the establishment of more formalised systems of health system governance. Specifically in relation to the activities of doctors, new institutional structures were introduced to more closely regulate their practice and to ensure that their professional concerns did not subvert the primary organisational goal of improving the performance of the health system. Looking back a decade on from the introduction of managerialism, Celia Davies argued that it represented the most fundamental challenge to the working practices of the health professions that had occurred in the then 60-year history of the NHS:

> For many people working inside the NHS, the early 1990s felt like a period of total revolution in health care. New vocabularies of business management pervaded thinking. Markets and managerialism came to the fore, and competition and contracting were the order of the day .... (however) the real revolution came later, after 1997, New Labour began not just to reshape once again the overall organisational arrangements of healthcare, but to redesign the workforce. Assumptions about the professional autonomy of doctors, about the hierarchies and divisions of labour between and among other health professions that had survived successive health service reorganisation's of earlier decades began to be cast aside.
>
> (Davies:2003;1)

Davies' statement proved to be prophetic. In 2007, legislation was introduced to fundamentally reform the GMC eding 150 years of self-regulation. But this reform process had been a long and drawn-out one. The introduction of the NPM was a major factor, but there were other considerations also in play. For many years, and well before the fiscal crises of the late 1970s, a political and institutional consensus had begun to emerge which recognised that the traditional oversight bodies (the 'trinity') were increasingly unworkable and untenable. In particular, the existing legal framework in relation to the civil liability of doctors in patient safety cases was deemed to be too deferential to the profession. Public confidence in this system of self-regulation had been undermined by the ineffective and slow response of the GMC in cases of individual underperformance and incompetence (McDonald:2012;98).

By the 1990s, a series of high-profile scandals had further heightened public concerns, forcing the government into setting-up a series of investigatory public inquiries to draw lessons that could be integrated into a future reform of the system of professional self-regulation. Thirteen public inquiries were held in the 13 years between 1992 and 2005, the majority of which involved substantial allegations of poor clinical performance and professional conduct. The UK government's eventual response, after failing to persuade the GMC to introduce its own internal reforms, was to publish a White Paper setting-out detailed proposals to ensure patient safety and quality of health care; this was entitled, *Trust, Assurance and Safety – The Regulation of Health Professionals in the 21st Century* (Secretary of State for Health:2007). This White Paper led onto primary legislation, the 2008 *Health and Social Care Act*, which brought about a fundamental restructuring of the GMC, including new 'fitness to practice' and associated re-validation arrangements for doctors. Non-medical lay members were now to constitute half of the GMC membership, and an independent system overseen by the Public Appointments Commission was introduced to elect these members. A new yardstick for the assessment of professional underperformance was established that moved away from the criminal law standard of 'beyond all reasonable doubt', so that the behaviour of doctors could now be judged on the civil standard of proof, 'on the balance of probability'. In summary, the effective ending of the relative autonomy of the medical profession and its integration into an overarching system of NHS governance represented the outcome of a combination of organisational and social structural changes emergent at the end of the twentieth century.

The NPM and health system governance – four decades on

The 'new' in 'NPM' is clearly no longer pertinent, but it is salient to assess the long-term impact of the re-organisation of health and welfare institutions in the UK and across European States nearly four decades on. In late 1980s, few of these governments were neoliberal in political orientation,[7] but nearly all were convinced that a fundamental re-orientation and structuring of public service organisation was required to bring about a much needed improvement in the quality, efficiency and effectiveness of public service provision. More recently, some commentators have talked in terms of the 'transcendence' of the NPM following a series of more reforms that have focused on improving the coordination, centralisation and collaborative capacity of public service organisations (Lægreid & Christensen:2017). But other analysts disagree and have argued that it is more accurate to talk about continuity rather than a shift away from core NPM organisational principles in public services. Lapuente and Vaan de Wale (2020) have made the point that: '(P)ost-NPM reforms do not substantially differ from NPM. They blend NPM aspects like marketisation and the use of NPM-style management tools with some neo-Weberian characteristics of bureaucracy such as a renewed emphasis on impartiality, or they build on some of the same elements complemented with the reintegrating tendencies offered by digital-era governance practices' (p464).

The five core characteristics of the NPM that discussed above are re-examined below in the context of subsequent developments in the management of public health and welfare services. The purpose being to determine whether it is possible to discern a 'continuity' of these characteristics in the structure, functioning, and culture of contemporary governance systems in the UK and across Europe. It should be noted that these organisational characteristics are analytical rather than empirical categories, so inevitably there will be a degree of overlap between each of them.

Incentivisation – four decades on

At the inception of the NPM, it was claimed that a 'results-orientated' approach would serve to incentivise the performance of employees as well as the organisation as a whole. This it was claimed, would be in contrast to the 'process-driven' routines of traditional bureaucratic authority, marked by rule-based hierarchies where obedience and aversion to risk-taking were culturally valued. Yet it was clear that this back-and-white contrast between bureaucratic and 'results-driven' forms of public organisation did not always reflect the empirical realities. An early cross-national European research study conducted a decade after these reforms had occurred appeared to demonstrate that in many cases the procedural bureaucratic rules of public sector management had not lessened with the introduction of NPM. Rather, it was the case that existing bureaucracies had been augmented with additional regulatory regimes of governance, described as a basic case of 'goal displacement' (Pollitt et al:1999).

Unlike private sector organisations from where the NPM drew its inspiration, public service institutions frequently have to deal with organisational goal ambiguities, in particular, responding to demands from public service users for more spending to improve the quality of a service, and from governments seeking to impose funding restrictions. These tensions necessarily complicate the construction of an incentive-based reward system for employees. Local health service managers, for example, have clear constraints on the scope of motivation-enhancing incentive measures that they may want to introduce. They cannot give their subordinates relative autonomy in the performance of their administrative roles if institutional responsibilities are mandated by legislation and subject to public accountability (Lapuente & Vaan de Wale:2020;465). The tax paying public and their elected representatives have a direct interest in holding public service institutions such as the NHS to higher ethical standards and closer scrutiny than they would private sector commercial services, such as mobile phone services or energy suppliers for example.

Bevan and Hood's (2006) study of the post-NPM behaviour of NHS institutions concluded that the attempts to incentivise meeting national performance targets simply resulted in an explosion of institutional 'gaming' behaviour. Here, incentivisation is seen to have had a significant negative long-term impact on the process of governance. In other cases, incentivisation has directly led onto employees prioritising the meeting of measurable output targets at the expense of fulfilling core public service duties, so they would receive rewards. When local health care trusts report that they have met their performance targets, neither government nor the public are in a position to be able to distinguish between the following possible outcomes. (a) All is well: performance has been exactly as desired whether measured or not. (b) The performance of the organisations has been as desired where it was measured, in the domains where it was not measured the potential for poor performance is high. (c) Organisational measurable performance is good, but its activities have been at variance with the substantive goals behind the health care targets; hitting targets but missing the point! (d) Performance targets have not been met, but this has been concealed by the way in which the data was reported or by outright fabrication (Bevan & Hood:2006;421).

Organisational gaming behaviour appears to have become more entrenched over the decades. More recent research by Lewis (2016) has pointed to some high-profile cases in health care organisations where seemingly positive outcomes on a range of performance indicators have been shown to mask overall sub-standard levels of care. Boruvka and Perry (2000) have also drawn attention to the long-term consequences of extrinsic incentives on the intrinsic motivations of individuals seeking employment within the public service sector: '(W)ith its emphasis on rewards and its neglect of altruism, NPM may have replaced "knights" for "knaves"' (p570). Furthermore, these same authors argue that efficiency and quality outcomes are not consistent one with the other, and this is because of the unpredictability of the outcomes of extrinsic incentivised rewards on employee behaviour.

Competition and marketisation – four decades on

The debate about the benefits or otherwise of introducing competition into the provision of public services continues to the present day. The original proponents of the NPM argued that the creation of a competitive market for service provision provided incentives for greater efficiency. However there is a counter-argument, and this is that the principle accountability of any private sectors provider is to their shareholders, not the public users of the service. Therefore, these providers have an incentive to reduce the quality of a service in order to cut costs and so increase profits, especially given that it is a much more straightforward process to measure the costs rather than the quality of service provision. Whatever position is adopted, creating a quasi-market that operates with the 'invisible hand' of competition has proven to be problematic. Internal service providers in the state health care sector, such as NHS hospitals, cannot be simply made bankrupt and go to the wall if they prove to be less than 'competitive'. Even the competition rules of the Thatcherite 'internal' market did not allow for this situation to occur, if they did then it would directly have ushered in full-scale privatisation of the NHS which would never had been acceptable to the British general public. While the terminology of 'competition' has been played down over the decades, the purchaser-provider separation continues and private sector companies continue to play an important role within the NHS.[8]

The procurement or 'commissioning' process that involves tendering for contracts to provide a public service should in principle be open and subject to public scrutiny. Information about a bidding company's performance record should be transparent, yet this is not always the case in both the UK and the EU despite the existence of legislation in both jurisdictions designed to prevent anti-competitive agreements and the abuse of a dominant market position: '(I)n the literature transparency is regarded as a purifying force of government. In the absence of transparent systems ... fraud and corruption can proliferate and competition is distorted' (Lapuente & Vaan de Wale:2020;469).

Disaggregation – four decades on

Disaggregation is a key NPM principle, linked to the facilitation of a competitive process for public service provision and marked by the ending of an aggregated funding and service delivery role for public service organisations. A process that become known as 'agentification' followed disaggregation, with public health service and social welfare organisations narrowing their remit and becoming solely purchaser's or 'commissioners' of public services.[9] One critical assessment of this process is that while public service agencies have seen a considerable expansion in their role in conducting audits and performance assessments of service providers, their role in collecting the data necessary to evaluate the outcomes of strategic policy programmes has not kept pace and has received nothing like the same level of institutional attention. By definition, health policy programmes necessarily extend beyond the confines of individual provider organisations, and the consequence of limited aggregated performance data has been that evidence-based policy-making has become much more problematic (Peters & Pierre:2020).

The role played by McKinsey, the global management consultancy company, in the process of disaggregation and marketisation of services in the NHS has been an interesting one. McKinsey and Co has been in the business of advising private and public companies how best to enhance their efficiency and maximise their profit margins since before the Second World War. The key elements that have long characterised the approach of McKinsey consultants when advising clients has been to reduce staff numbers, increase the productivity of those remaining, and outsource (and offshore) work to contractors where possible in order to reduce costs and raise profitability. McKinsey consultants offer their services in all sectors of the global economy, from large manufacturing companies to service sector clients. They have for many years been embedded in the US health care system, advising private health insurance companies, as well as the state-aided Medicaid insurance scheme.

The NPM re-organisation in the late 1980s was the opportunity for management consultancies such as McKinsey to offer their services advising government about how best to set about the process of marketising service provision, and in its wake open doors to private sector service operator's, including US companies to enter the NHS system. By 2010, as a newly elected Conservative government was preparing the ground for a further re-organisation of the NHS, McKinsey consultants were in prime position given their long-standing association with several senior politicians as well as health officials to advise on a new phase of the commissioning process. The 2012 *The Health and Social Care Act* gave commissioning powers to primary care doctors via newly created local Clinical Commissioning Groups (CCGs), which were now to be held responsible for the majority of the NHS spending budget.[10] Section 75 of this legislation required CCGs to ensure that all their service provision contracts were open to tender. However, these doctor-led CCGs had little or no experience of tendering and commissioning services, McKinsey consultants were to play a prominent role in the £7 million contract that was awarded to advise these groups (Bogdanich & Forsythe:2022;272). The 2012 legislation also saw a new high point in the share of NHS funding awarded to private sector companies for clinical and other patient services. A decade later, the system was to be restructured yet again, and the local commissioning CCGs were replaced with yet another iteration of the agentification process, this time in the form of regional Integrated Care Board's (ICB).[11]

A further example of McKinsey's closeness to government health decision-making occurred during the 2020 pandemic. In Bogdanich and Forsythe's polemical 'exposé', *When McKinsey Comes to Town* (2022), the authors relate the situation when Prime Minister Boris Johnson entrusted the all-important COVID-19 test-and-trace effort to the former McKinsey consultant Dido Harding, now Baroness Harding; '(S)he and the country's top health officials turned to private companies, not the NHS, to run the program. McKinsey alone charged £563,400 to provide a "vision, purpose and narrative" of the Harding-led program' (p274).

Measurable system outputs – four decades on

Two decades ago, Hood and Peters (2004) identified a number of what they termed 'paradoxes' associated with the development of performance output indicators.[12] They argued that measuring the performance of the health care system was not a straightforward process, care delivery could not be treated as a pure process of 'production' in the same way that commercial companies utilise commodity output measures. Yet this concern has not prevented the development of a range of indices to assess service provider quality of care, efficiency, and effectiveness of interventions. The question of whether these indicators were able to effectively embrace the complexity and nuances of health system functionality, for example in assessing whether quality improvement interventions effectively took account of pre-existing health inequities, was one that was either absent or relegated to the margins of organisational performance assessment (Nundy et al:2022;521).

The organisation of work – four decades on

As previously described, a substantial programme reconfiguring professional roles and responsibilities followed in the wake of the initial NPM re-structuring of the NHS. One illustrative case demonstrates some of the ways in which this process had unanticipated consequences for the quality of patient health care. In 2003, a new clinical role was introduced within the NHS, that of the Physicians Associate (PA). The role of the PA was first developed in the US health care system in the 1960s and was originally designed to free-up doctors from having to undertake routinised tasks so that they could utilise their expertise (as well as their time) more effectively. In England, PAs undertake two years of training at either undergraduate or postgraduate level, but they qualify as generalists who do not have a medical degree so are unable to prescribe medications. PAs constitute part of the multidisciplinary clinical team, but they are required to work under the close supervision of a named senior doctor (Royal College of Physicians:2024). Although initially welcomed, the PA role has more recently produced a backlash amongst many doctors working in the NHS who have become concerned that a blurring of professional boundaries is now occurring. There is also a concern that doctors are now witnessing an increase rather than decrease in the amount of clinical time they are having to spend supervising PAs as the numbers have expanded over time.[13] The paradox here is that that despite the development of governance systems regulating medical professional practice, an equivalent oversight of PAs does not appear to have kept pace with changing working practices. These concerns have become increasingly prominent following a number of high-profile cases of unsupervised PAs misdiagnosing or mismanaging patients.

There is a well-established history of the study of the consequences of a whole-sale restructuring of roles in the workplace, the lessons of which seemed to have been ignored or elided during the implementation of the NPM reforms. Harry Braverman's (1974) classic study of corporate America in the 1970s, subtitled 'The degradation of work in the Twentieth Century', describes how changes in industrial production led onto a process of deskilling, rationalisation, and a degradation of established work roles and responsibilities. Management consultants, including McKinsey (discussed above), had played a significant role in advising employers on how best to cut labour costs and improve efficiency and productivity. As described by Braverman, this 'degradation of work' was a process that impacted at all levels of a workforce, from unskilled to pro-fessional occupations, deepening dissatisfaction and alienating the existing workforce. Although this study was written over half-a-century ago and was focused mainly on the manufacturing industry, in many ways its conclusions could also apply to the out-comes of the re-organisation of work roles within the health and welfare services in the UK and beyond.

In 2024, a wave of national strikes occurred amongst professional staff working in the NHS, including doctors, nurses, and physiotherapists. The key issues for these health care staff were increased workload, low pay, and a reduction in the resources necessary to meet their professional responsibilities to patient management and care. In recent years, strikes of doctors and nurses have also occurred in Italy, France, and Germany for many of the same reasons. The relative loss of professional status and decision-making autonomy, associated with a managerialist rationalising and techni-cising of professional roles, has led onto the situation where any appeals to a 'service ethic' in support of an under-funded system are increasingly falling on deaf ears. Many health care professionals today would all too readily recognise the processes associated with the 'degradation' of their working lives now manifest in the twenty-first century within the public service sector.

A decentralised or centralised system of health system governance?

Traditional state bureaucratic systems of command-control governance are character-ised by clear lines of authority and communication. But in the post-NPM period, many policy analysts have argued that the control once exerted by central government in relation to the state provision of health services has been effectively 'hollowed-out'. Alternatively it has been argued that we should now think in terms of a decentralised state health care system, 'where the executive decides the What, but the How is in the hands of autonomous agencies whose managers have incentives to deliver in the most efficient ways' (Lapuente & Vaan de Wale:2020;471).

In 1990, new delegated powers were granted to the regional and local levels of the health care system in England, over the course of the following decades the issue of where the balance of public accountability lies in relation to the functioning and effi-ciency of the NHS in England. With Ministers of State? the civil service functioning within a Ministry of Health? with arms-length bodies such as NHS England? with the disaggregated semi-autonomous regional and local health care commissioning agen-cies? or with the proliferation of autonomous service delivery organisations? In sim-plified terms, who exactly is accountable to the public for ensuring that the national health service delivers on its overarching mission, ensuring sustainable universal health care provision that equitably meets population health needs? Have the processes associated with 'decentralisation' advanced to such a degree that there is now a clear risk of the national health system fragmenting?

One of the 'paradox's' of the NPM re-organisation of the health care system, as identified by Hood and Peters (2004), it was initially hoped that the transfer of direct responsibility for day-to-day service delivery away from formal government control, was an effective method of 'de-politicising' the health system. No more would government Ministers of State have to stand up in Parliament and directly address tricky and embarrassing questions about the performance of the NHS. In practice what occurred was an increase in the incidence of politicians having to intervene in the appointment (or sacking) of managers in arms-length health care bodies, in order for government to retain some semblance of control over the implementation of their health policies.

The COVID-19 pandemic brought these matters to a head. A decentralised response to a global pandemic was never going to end well, and in the UK as well as throughout Europe, governments intervened to take back centralised control, in order to be able to formulate and implement an effective and coordinated national strategic response. The much-vaunted efficiency of the NPM regime that saw a reduction over the decades in the numbers of hospital bed and facilities in the NHS as a cost-saving process, meant that when the pandemic arrived there was not the flexibility within the system to meet the challenge of the pandemic. There was now a requirement for specialised intensive care facilities, as well as sufficient beds within hospitals to transfer patients to when the most intensive period of their treatment was complete. This led to the appalling situation whereby patients who were still receiving medical treatment were transferred from hospitals to residential and nursing care homes as there was no where else for them to go. Here staff had neither the training nor protective equipment to prevent the spread of the virus, leading directly to a disproportionate number of deaths of the elderly residents of these homes directly due to their exposure to the virus.

Governments across Europe 'took back a great deal of control at the expense of autonomous agencies in the context of the 2020 pandemic and gave orders where they might previously have tried to steer systems through contracts, competition, or regulations. In some cases, such as England, that recentralisation may last' (Greer et al:2021;39). This conjecture was made in 2021, and in 2022 the NHS in England did indeed undergo an organisational reform (*The Health and Care Act*). Although this was not a re-centralisation of strategic and funding decision-making at the national level, it did embrace a re-integration of structures of decision-making at the regional level in England.

The governance of resource priority-setting

One of the key roles played by structures of governance in public services is to 'optimise' the utilisation of funding resources so as to ensure equity of provision. This is a dimension of policy-making that has been widely termed 'priority-setting' or more colloquially as 'rationing'. Since the inception of post-war publically-funded universal health care systems the question of how to square the circle of an ever-increasing demand for health care with finite health spending resources has been ever present. Political and social tensions inevitable arise when the necessity of determining spending priorities comes into conflict with socially normative expectations concerning the availability and provision of health care. Generally speaking, the formal process of health resource priority-setting[14] follow a set of bureaucratic decision-rules, this is process is known as 'consequentialism'. However, the public policy literature also recognises an alternative approach that has been adopted in some health systems. This is known by the term 'proceduralism' and is so named as it aims to enhance a direct stakeholder (citizens/patients) engagement in the setting of resource priority criteria.

Consequentialist forms of priority-setting governance

In theory, consequentialism should follow a formal and explicit set of criteria ('instrumental justification') to guide the distribution of health resources. However, given that priority-setting is unavoidably a value-laden process, it is perhaps unsurprising that explicit details of the criteria that are used to ration health care resources in the NHS remain somewhat elusive.[15] This reticence almost certainly reflects a concern to avoid any potential for politicising a process that health officials would rather remain bureaucratic and opaque. Nevertheless, there are several key evaluative criteria that feature prominently in academic discussions of the prioritising of public service resources. These typically include the categories of efficiency, effectiveness, and cost-effectiveness.[16] While the application of the principle of equity should ideally mean that, 'decisions are generally fairest when standards are predetermined, explicit and consistently applied' (Guindo:2012;10).

Unlike NHS England, several European health care systems have been quite explicit about the use of consequentialist priority-setting criteria to determine resource allocation for patient treatment. The Norwegian government established an independent commission to establish principles for prioritisation in the late 1980s. This body determined that severity of medical condition was the only basis for prioritising of treatment. A decade later, now firmly within the NPM era, cost-effectiveness of treatment was added as a further consideration. In the Netherlands in the 1990s, an independent advisory committee was established in order to determine a set of criteria for the treatment of patients. The criteria that were chosen lacked specificity but included necessity, effectiveness, efficiency, and personal responsibility. Sweden adopted a very similar approach when it established a parliamentary priorities commission in the early 1990s. This body eventually recommended four rather less than clinically specific principles to be utilised in the process of prioritising health resources; human dignity, health need, solidarity, and cost-efficiency. But it was also specified that these four criteria were to be used only in comparing treatments for the same condition. In 1996, the Danish Council of Ethics, an independent body established in 1988 to provide the Danish Parliament, local authorities, as well as the public with advice and information concerning ethical problems, set out four key principles for prioritising health care treatment. These principles were equality, solidarity, security, and autonomy (Sabik & Lie:2008). While the governance arrangements for setting criteria for treatment priority have been transparent in these four countries, it is all but impossible to translate these criteria into the accounting language of NPM health service commissioning, nor do they translate well at the level of the clinical management of individual patients.

Proceduralist forms of priority-setting governance

Proceduralism is a deliberative approach to priority-setting that seeks to determine health resource allocation through processes of public engagement, with the objective of ascertaining which health care priorities best meet the values or principles shared by a particular community (Mooney:2005). One frequently cited example of this stakeholder-focused approach occurred in Oregon State (in the USA) in the early 1990s. It was at this time that the State of Oregon made the decision to extend the coverage of the Medicaid health care insurance program[17] to 100% (from 58%) for all those living below the federal poverty line, but without increasing the overall Medicaid budget. The proposal was to fund the programme by restricting free care to a bundle of services known as the 'Health Plan'. To determine which treatments were to be included and which excluded in the 'bundle', a ranking scale of available treatments was drawn up and subjected to a process of public consultation that involved public hearings, town hall meetings and a telephone survey. This approach was ultimately abandoned following a massive public outcry. The citizens of Oregon essentially rejected the imposition of a process that required them to decide which clinical treatment should be made available and which not, to the most vulnerable members of their communities. Over a decade later in 2003, the State of Oregon tried again, but this time they utilised a consequentialist approach. They established an expert commission (similar to those described above existing in Scandinavian countries) to rank health care services that would be available to those on Medicaid on the basis of more abstract criteria discussed above (Perry & Hotze:2011).

Other than the State of Oregon 'experiment', there are few other substantive examples of community stakeholder involvement in the process of governance in order to determine health resource priority-setting. However, there have been attempts in the Netherlands to establish a community stakeholder consensus around health policy-agenda setting and resource prioritisation. This approach is known as the 'Dialogue Model' and has been adopted in a number of cases involving specific patient community's and local citizen forums over the past decade (Schölvinck et al:2020;248). The position of the Dutch Ministry of Health is that these small-scale examples of stakeholder involvement provide some legitimacy to its own centralised consequentialist priority-setting process. One recent study provides an insightful qualitative analysis of one of these deliberative citizen forum's in action (Jansen et al:2022). The study looked at whether the views of individual forum participants changed when they engaged in the process of jointly deciding which clinical treatments or interventions should be subject to the reimbursement of patients' health costs. Noting that in the Dutch social insurance system not all basic medical costs are reimbursed because of Health Care budget limits. The study reached the conclusion that: '(P)roviding opportunities for critical deliberation is key to prevent citizens from adhering to initial emotional reactions that remain unchallenged and which may no longer be supported after deliberation' (Jansen et al:2022;126). Whether the Dutch Ministry of Health has taken on board these findings in its own centralised priority-setting is a moot point.

Concluding comments

The concept of governance, in the analytical context of the institutions of accountability operating within a national health system, offers a schematic understanding of the processes that are in strategic decision-making, resource allocation, and the regulation of activities within a system of health care. Yet, the application of the governance heuristic should not be read as alternative to a power analysis.[18] Despite the proliferation of arms-length and autonomous bodies with responsibilities for the commissioning and provision of health care for the population of England, it remains the case, that the authority for setting the legislative, regulatory, and funding constraints on the health care system continues to reside with the elected central government. Systems of governance change over time, but the fiscal restraints and top-down priorities imposed on these bodies since the late 1980s remain.

Notes

1 These developments were not by chance strongly connected to the emergence of neoliberal economic state policies in many Western countries at the time – described in Chapter 1.
2 This concept is described in detail in Chapter 1
3 See discussion on path-dependency in Chapter 2.
4 Weber's equally influential work on Bureaucracy as well as his work on Authority was discussed in Chapter 2.
5 The analytical approach to policy development known as 'historical institutionalism' was discussed in Chapter 2.
6 This process is described in detail in Chapter 7.
7 Dissatisfaction with the performance of state bureaucracies in the delivery of public services was not limited to the political 'right'. Scandinavian social democratic governments were also responsible for introducing some elements of NPM into their own public services.
8 Discussed in detail in Chapter 7.
9 See Figure 7.2 and Figure 7.3 in Chapter 7, which schematically represents the commissioning roles of health service organisation in both the YK and Germany, respectively.
10 The 2012 re-organisation and the role of CCGs are discussed in Chapter 7.
11 The 2020 re-organisation and the role of ICBs are discussed in Chapter 7.
12 Health system indicators of performance are discussed in relation to comparative analysis in Chapter 5.
13 In March 2024, the UK government announced it wanted to increase the number of PAs working in the NHS, from 3200 in 2024 to 10,000 by 2036.
14 The policy decision-making process is the subject of Chapter 2.
15 One recent example of this reticence can be seen in a document published by the NHS England, the purpose of which is to provide post-COVID priority-setting planning guidance for managers for operational purposes. But where it might be expected that explicit criteria would be found, these are referred to only in very generalised terms (NHS:2022).
16 These categories are assessed in detail in the context of output-orientated comparative system analysis in Chapter 5.
17 Medicaid is a joint federal and state government funded programme that provides health care insurance for adults and families with below average incomes. The US government sets a baseline standard for state Medicaid programmes, but there is a considerable range of eligibility found across the 50 US states.
18 See Chapter 2 for a detailed appraisal of power analysis in the policymaking process.

References

Bevan, G and Hood, C (2006) Have targets improved performance in the English NHS? *British Medical Journal*, vol. 332, 419–422.

Bogdanich, W and Forsythe, M (2022) *When McKinsey Comes to Town*. London. The Bodley Head.

Boruvka, E and Perry, J (2020) Understanding evolving public motivational practices: an institutional analysis, *Governance*, vol. 33, no. 3, 565–584.

Braverman, H (1974) *Labor and Monopoly Capital: The Degradation of Work in the Twentieth Century*. London. Monthly Review Press.

Clarke, J (1998) 'Thriving on chaos? Managerialisation and social welfare', in Carter, J (ed) *Postmodernity and the Fragmentation of Welfare*. London. Routledge, pp 171–187.

Clarke, J (2004) *Changing Welfare, Changing States: New Directions in Social Policy*. London. Sage.

Davies, C (2003) 'Introduction: a new workforce in the making?' in Davies, C (ed) *The Future Health Workforce*. Basingstoke. Palgrave, pp 1–13.

Davies, W (2022) Madmen economics, *London Review of Books*, vol. 44, no. 20, 3–5.

Davies, C, Arnand, P, Holloway, J, McConway, K, Newman, J, Story, J and Thompson, G (2005) *Links between Governance Incentives and Outcomes: A Review of the Literature*. Report for the *National Coordinating Centre for the Service Delivery and Organisation*. Report for the National Co-ordinating Centre for NHS Service Delivery and Organisation. R&D (NCCSDO).

Dunleavy, P, Margetts, H, Bastow, S and Tinkler, J (2006) New Public Management is dead – long live digital era governance, *Journal of Public Administration Research and Theory*, vol. 16, no. 3, 467–494.

Friedson, E (1970) *The Profession of Medicine*. London. University of Chicago Press.

Greer, S, Falkenbach, M, Jarman, H, Löblavá, O, Rozenblum, S, Williams, N and Wismar, M (2021) Centralisation and decentralisation in a crises: how credit and blame shape governance, *Eurohealth*, vol. 27, no. 1, 36–40.

Greer, S, Wismar, M and Figueras, M (2016) 'Introduction: strengthening governance amidst changing governance' in Greer, S, Wismar, M and Figueras, M (eds) *Strengthening Health System Governance*. European Observatory on Health Systems and Policies. Maidenhead. Bucks Open University Press, pp 3–26.

Guindo, L, Wagner, M, Baltussen, R, Rindress, D, Van til, J, Kind, P and Goetghebeur, M (2012) From efficacy to equity: literature review of decision criteria for resource allocation and healthcare decision making, *Cost Effectiveness and Resource Allocation*, vol. 10, no. 9, 1–13.

Hill, M and Hupe, P (2014) *Implementing Public Policy* (3rd Ed). London. Sage.

Hood, C and Peters, B (2004) The middle ageing of new public management: into the age of paradox, *Journal of Public Administration Research and Theory*, vol. 14, no. 3, 267–282.

Hood, C and Scott, C (2000) *Regulating Government in a 'Managerial' Age: Towards a Cross-National Perspective*. London. Centre for Analysis of Risk and Regulation, LSE.

International Labour Office (2012) *International Standard Classification of Occupations ISCO-8*. Geneva, Switzerland. ILO.

Jansen, M, Baltussen, R, Bijlmakers, L and Tummers, M (2022) The Dutch Citizen Forum on public reimbursement of healthcare: a qualitative analysis of opinion change, *International Journal of Health Policy and Management*, vol. 11, no. 2, 118–127.

Lægreid, P and Christensen, T (2017) *Transcending New Public Management*. London. Routledge.

Lapuente, V and Van de Walle, S (2020) The effects of new public management on the quality of public services, *Governance: An International Journal of Policy, Administration and Institutions*, vol. 33, no. 3, 461–475.

Lewis, J (2016) 'The paradox of health care performance measurement and management' in Ferlie, K, Montgomery, K and Pedersen, A (eds) *The Oxford Handbook of Health Care Management*. Oxford. Oxford University Press, pp 375–392.

McDonald, F (2012) 'Challenging the regulatory trinity', in Short, S and McDonald, F (eds) *Health Workforce Governance: Improved Access, Good Regulatory Practice, Safer Patients*. Farnham. Ashgate, pp 97–112.

Mooney, G (2005) Communitarian claims and community responsibilities: furthering priority-setting? *Social Science and Medicine*, vol. 60, 247–255.

Moran, M (1999) *Governing the Health Care State*. Manchester. Manchester University Press.

Moran, M (2004) 'Governing doctors in the British Regulatory State', in Gray, A and Harrison, S (eds) *Governing Medicine; Theory and Practice* Maidenhead. Open University Press, pp 27–36.

Newman, J (2001) *Modernising Governance*. London. Sage.

NHS England (2022) *2022/23 Priorities and Operational Planning Guidance* (V3, February 2022). London. NHS England & NHS Improvement.

Nundy, S, Cooper, L and Mate, K (2022) The quintuple aim for health care improvement: a new imperative to advance health equity, *JAMA*, vol. 327, no. 6, 521–522.

Perry, P and Hotze, T (2011) Oregon's experiment with prioritizing public health care services, *American Medical Association Journal of Ethics*, vol. 13, no. 4, 241–247.

Peters, BG and Pierre, J (2020) From evaluation to auditing and from programs to institutions: causes and consequences of the decline of the program approach, *Governance*, vol. 33, no. 3, 585–597.

Pollitt, C, Girre, X, Lonsdale, J, Mul, R, Summa, H and Waerness, M (1999) *Performance or Compliance: Performance Audit and Public Management in Five Countries*. Oxford. Oxford University Press.

Pollitt, C, van Thiel, S and Homburg, V (2007) New Public Management in Europe. *Management Online Review*. October 2007.

Royal College of Physicians (2024) *Who Are Physician Associates?* https://fparcp.co.uk (accessed 05/2024).

Sabik, L and Lie, R (2008) Priority setting in health care: lessons from the experiences of eight countries, *International Journal for Equity in Health*, vol. 7, no. 4, 1–13.

Saks, M (2012) Defining a profession: the role of knowledge and expertise, *Professions and Professionalism*, vol. 2, no. 1, 1–10.

Schölvinck, A-F, Pittens, C and Broerse, J (2020) Patient involvement in agenda-setting processes in health research policy, *Science and Public Policy*, vol. 47, no. 2, 246–255.

Secretary of State for Health (2007) *Trust, Assurance and Safety – The Regulation of Health Professionals in the 21st Century* (White Paper – Cm 7013). London. The Stationary Office.

The funding and financing of health care systems

The funding and financing distinction

In public policy analysis, the terms 'funding' and 'financing' are frequently used interchangeably, but perhaps even more surprisingly, this is often the case in the world of banking too. But strictly speaking, the process of 'funding' is the act of *providing* money or capital for a given purpose, while 'financing' is the act of *receiving* money or capital for the purchasing of services or commodities. Drawing a distinction may initially appear to be pedantic, but an analytical separation enables a degree of clarity, particularly in the case of health care provision.

In those countries with state or public health system, the *financing* of health care provision comes either through a direct process of central government spending allocations or an indirect process of payment transfers from the central government to regional or local authorities. In these systems, the sources of *funding* are of three main kinds. Either direct taxation levied on income, wealth, and capital gains, compulsory social insurance deducted at source from wages, or alternatively some sort of hypothecated tax system.

In countries with predominately private health care systems, *financing* of health care provision mainly comes through private health insurance (PHI) companies. The *fund*s drawn upon by these PHI companies largely derives from the premiums paid by individual policy-holders, which, after a profitable margin has been extracted, is transferred to health care providers. In turn, the funding of the health care providers comes not only from extracting a percentage profit from the money transferred from the PHI companies, but also the financial markets, where shares are bought and traded, constituting the equity of these private health care providers.

The analytical separation of the financing from the funding of health care is reflected in the separate discussion sections within this chapter. Yet it should also be acknowledged that funding and financing health care is much messier in reality than a neat analytical separation might imply. The oscillations of state fiscal policy and the economy inevitably impact on government health care spending, particularly in those systems such as the National Health Service (NHS) which are funded through direct taxation. Even in those countries where universal health provision is funded through workplace-based social insurance payments, state fiscal policy and the relative performance of the economy directly effects the ability to maintain the required levels of social insurance payments and funding, dependant as they are on high levels of employment.

DOI: 10.4324/9781003564249-6

An outline of functional structures of financing and funding

In an analysis published by the World Health Organisation (WHO), Kutzin et al (2017) set out three core principles that they recommend should guide the functioning of any system of health care financing and funding.

(a) *Revenue raising*: Identifying the source of potential funding such as state budgets, external international aid, out-of-pocket payments made by users, and compulsory or voluntary contributions made by individuals via various insurance schemes. The WHO guiding principles are that health systems should 'move towards a predominant reliance on public/compulsory funding sources i.e. some form of taxation', in order to increase the predictability and the stability of funding over an extended period of years.

(b) *Pooling*: The primary function of any system of pooling is to, 'enhance the redistributive capacity of available prepaid funds (which in turn should) ... reduce fragmentation, duplication and overlap'.

(c) *Purchasing*: The allocation of monies and resources to provider organisations for the provision and delivery of health care services. The guiding principle for this system function is that it should seek to, 'increase the extent to which the allocation of resources to providers is linked to the health needs of the population they serve'. This in turn is seen to require systems to generate more accurate 'information on health service provider performance' in meeting these needs.

(Kutzin et al:2017;11–12)

At this point it be should be noted that the actual scope and content of financing and funding will inevitably differ as between high-, medium-, and low income countries[1] (HIC, MIC, LIC). It should further be noted that the WHO guidance follows the analytical distinction drawn above between the funding and financing of health care provision.

Having an effective system of pooling health care funds is generally seen to be a minimum requirement for achieving equitable health care provision in any given country in accordance with the United Nations Sustainable Development Goals (SDG's)[2]. Without such a system, the individual financial burden of paying for health care treatment would be considerable and in many cases completely unaffordable for families. Whether pooling of funds is achieved through some form of direct taxation on income), indirect taxation or goods purchased, or compulsory contribution to a health insurance scheme, the cost-related risks attached to becoming unwell and requiring treatment can be shared across a large number of people. However, there are some forms of health care cost pooling, such as private insurance schemes, which necessarily exclude those deemed to be 'risks', that is those individuals already in poor health so likely to incur higher spending by the PHI scheme to health care service providers. Furthermore, not all compulsory health insurance schemes are able fully meet all the costs of treatment, so necessitating additional out-of-pocket payments (OOP).

Global trends in health system financing

Public spending constituted 44.8% UK GDP in 2023–24, although this proportional share is forecast to decline over the next five years (OBR:2023;93). The State in the UK raises the funds it requires to finance public spending through a combination of taxation

(£1,098 billion) and public sector borrowing (£123 billion), the latter secured through the international financial markets. Income tax and National Insurance Contributions represent approximately a third of all public sector receipts, with the remainder derived from VAT, Corporation tax, and various other regressive taxes. The state spends these monies on the day-to-day costs of providing public services (including health care), on capital investment, and on cash transfer payments to support the incomes of individuals and families.

Public spending in all four of the constituent countries of the UK is subject to limits set by the Treasury, the government's economic and finance ministry. In the financial year 2023–24, the Office of Budget Responsibility forecast that public spending would amount to £1,222 billion. This total public spend is broken down as follows: the largest single item was welfare spending on social security and tax credits at £295 billion, of which some £125 billion went to state pension payments and £77 billion on universal credit payments. The next single biggest item was government departmental spending representing £426 billion of the total. The three largest spending departments are Health and Social care – £175 billion; Education – £76 billion; and Defence – £32 billion (OBR:2023;98). The UK government generates less revenue relative to national income than Scandinavian countries but more than in the USA, Japan, and Korea. While public sector spending as a share of national income in the UK is slightly above the average of other OECD HIC's, but less than Finland or France (OECD:2022).

In 2020, global health spending[3] amounted to some US$9 trillion or 10.8% of global GDP. HIC's accounted for about 80% of this spending (with the USA alone accounting for 43.5%), despite accounting for only 15.3% of the world's population. Upper-MICs with 33% of the world's population, accounted for 16% of global spending, and lower-MICs with 43% of the world's population, just under 4% of spending. But of the greatest concern is the situation that pertains in LICs with 8% of the world's population who collectively spend just 0.2% of the global total (WHO:2022;2).

The trend in health spending (measured as a percentage of GDP) across these four income groupings for the period 2000–20 is shown in Figure 4.1. Average spending increased across all income classifications during this period, but spending rose most rapidly in HICs (2.7% on average), while LICs experienced just a 1% increase. The dip or flattening of health spending following the 2008 global fiscal crises should be noted, although the COVID-19 pandemic resulted in significant increases in spending across all income groups from 2020. This increase was most notable in LICs, where health spending as a percentage of GDP rose by an average of 18.6% in 2020, up to US$9.20 per capita. However, this rise was from a very low spending base level. In HICs by contrast, average spending as a percentage of GDP rose by 11.0%, equivalent to US$2,689 per capita!

Looking in more detail at the impact of the COVID-19 pandemic, in most HICs and LICs where enforced 'lockdowns' were imposed, a slowdown in the economy then occurred that in turn reduced public tax receipts. In these countries, the increase in health care spending did not result from economic growth (as was the case in the period 2000–2019), but reflected an increase in public borrowing in order to cover the gap from falling tax revenues. Also in many cases, public sector borrowing was combined

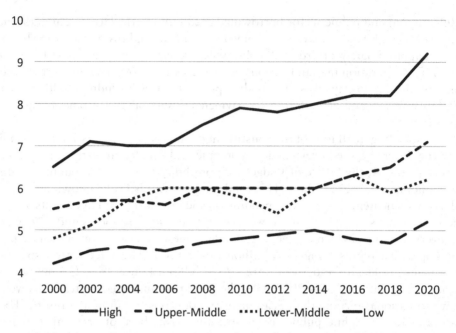

Figure 4.1 Health spending as percentage (%) of GDP: high-, upper-middle, lower-middle, and low-income countries 2000–20 (Adapted from WHO (2023)).

with redistribution policies that were weighting heavily towards public health interventions (WHO:2022;5).

Figure 4.2 shows public spending on health as a percentage of total government budget spending over a period of two decades, from 2000 to 2018 (noting that 2018 was chosen as the end point of the timeline, as year-on-year comparisons become difficult after this point following the significant increase in health spending in all countries during the COVID 19 pandemic). Many MICs and LICs also saw an increase in public spending on health care in this period. However, as noted by the World Health Organisation, these countries also '(N)eed to pay attention to reducing out-of-pocket payments to counter unmet need for health and dental care and financial hardship for people using health services. Both of these negative outcomes disproportionately affect poorer households and other groups of people in vulnerable situations' (WHO Regional Office for Europe:2021;xv).

The historical trends in health spending within HICs is set out in Figure 4.3. The timeline begins in 1960, which is essentially the point at which national universal health care systems were being consolidated within six of the countries shown, although not the USA where the private sector has always dominated. The chart demonstrates that while there was some disparity in spending levels as a percentage of GDP in 1960, ranging from around 3% to nearly 6%, all seven countries experienced a gradual real terms increase over the following four decades. This growth is commensurate with the real terms expansion of these economies over this time period, although the US health care system is clearly an outlier.

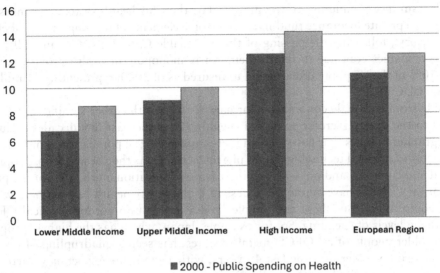

Figure 4.2 Public spending on health (% of government spending) by country income classification + WHO European Region (Adapted from WHO Regional Office for Europe (2021)).

However, identifying a correlation between the rise in health care spending as a percentage of GDP and the rate of economic growth in a given country is somewhat simplistic. Nor should it be assumed that a rise in health spending equates to an expansion in the quality and provision of health services in a given country. For example, although there was an exponential increase in health spending in the USA post-1970s, this rise is generally attributed to the additional costs that accrue in a predominantly private market system, including widening profit margins and increases in

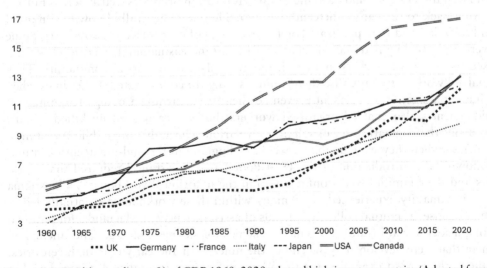

Figure 4.3 Health spending as % of GDP 1960–2020 selected high-income countries (Adapted from OECD (1989, 2022)).

health insurance premiums. To the present day, the USA health system continues its reliance on private insurance funding, even if some elements of funding can be labelled 'compulsory', following the passing of the Affordable Care Act (ACA) in 2010. For profit companies continue to retain their nearly monopoly of health provision, and some 10% of the US population remain uninsured as of 2020, representing 31 million people (CDC:2022).

Aside from national economic performance, some of the other significant factors linked to the steady increase in health spending over the past few decades include: demographic changes that have seen an increasing ageing of populations; an increase in the cost of medical technologies and pharmaceuticals as they become more sophisticated and complex; and not least, an increasing expectation on the part of the public that they should have automatic access to high-quality health care services when they require them. But these are complex processes and do not automatically lead onto rising levels of spending. So, for example, Japan, which has the highest proportion of older people of all OECD member states, has seen a quadrupling of people aged 65 years or older over the last 40 years, with average life expectancy currently at 85 years of age. Yet health spending in Japan, measured as a proportion of GDP, is far from being the highest of the seven countries shown in Figure 4.3. This is at least partially explained by the quality of social care and support provided for older citizens. Japan is committed to maintaining the independence of its older citizens for as long as possible.[4] Measuring health care spending only in terms of % GDP is also analytically problematic, and a further illustration of the importance of separating the assessment of the financing from the funding of health care provision in any given country.

Health care funding types

The earliest examples of national resource 'pooling' for the collective funding of health and welfare services could be found in various forms in Britain as well as across Europe dating back to the early nineteenth century. They were generally known as 'mutual aid societies' and were predicated on the principles of reciprocity and solidarity. Some were organised by paternalistic charities, but an increasing number were self-organised by groups of workers in a particular workplace or in a local community. They enabled workers to mutualise their limited savings to compensate for the times when illness, old age, or an accident prevented them from earning a living. These mutual aid schemes also enabled organised workers (but not casualised unskilled labour) to avoid the stigmatisation of reliance on various charitable or 'Public Assistance' schemes when they were unable to work. In England in the mid-nineteenth century, following the introduction of the 1834 Poor Laws, 'assistance' required that workers and their families were confined within the notorious 'workhouses'. The stigma and inhumanity experienced by so many within these workhouses eventually led to their demise, as mutual collectivist forms of assistance became the model for national compulsory social insurance payment schemes for sickness, old age, and unemployment that were developed at the end of the nineteenth and early twentieth centuries. One of the earliest examples was the *Workers Sickness Insurance Act* introduced in

1883 in the newly unified Germany under the chancellorship of Otto Von Bismarck.[5] In Britain, the Health Insurance Act was enacted in 1911 and covered a wider range of employed industrial workers (although their families and the unwaged were not covered by the scheme).

Freeman (2000;17) has asserted that the emergence of these statutory social insurance schemes reflected the interrelated processes of industrialisation and democratisation. The extension of the franchise to adult males (women would be made to wait much longer for the franchise to be extended to them) in Britain and elsewhere in Europe, meant that governments were now having to respond to democratic pressure for welfare reform. Voting rights was one factor, but crucially this was combined with an increasing number of industrial workers joining organised trade unions who were prepared to take action in support of demands for greater job security and welfare rights. Western Europe saw an incremental expansion of health insurance schemes extending sickness cover to the majority of the working (but not unwaged) population over the course of the early twentieth century. What emerged was array of social health insurance (SHI) schemes. Some of these SHI schemes operated through the private market, some were charitable, and some were examples of mutual aid. As such they provided welfare insurance cover for a range of social and occupational groups, involving local, regional, as well as national governments in administrative oversight roles. This mélange of provision, with many unskilled and informal workers having little or no possibility of joining an SHI, was inefficient and so unsustainable.

The post-war development of 'welfare states'[6] saw the introduction of universal health and welfare coverage for populations for the first time, funded through statutory health insurance health or through direct taxation. Today, there are only two countries in Europe, the Netherlands, and Switzerland, which organise compulsory funding through PHI schemes additional to SHI schemes. Outside of Europe, Canada provides an example of another method of funding, hypothecated direct tax, a form of block funding of health care. PHI continues to be the predominate form of funding in the USA, as it also is in many medium- and low-income countries where UHC is not an entitlement. Each of these funding systems is outlined in detail below.

Social health insurance

The founding principles of social solidarity that led on to the development of 'sickness insurance funds' today constitutes the basis of UHC and 'social protection' rights in countries with SHI-funded national welfare states. A typical SHI scheme provides cover for a defined package of health and welfare services, with employee contributions generally matched by that of their employers. As of 2021, 17 countries in the WHO European Region have compulsory SHI funding schemes (WHO Regional Office for Europe:2021;33). SHI funding schemes also serve as the preponderant source of funding for health care in the majority of upper-middle-income countries across the globe (WHO Regional Office for Europe;2021;36). Although there is considerable diversity in the structures and organisation of these systems, the ethos that they have in common is that they are; 'stable, tradition-bound social institution in which economic implications play an important role but do not exercise primary influence over decision-making' (Saltman:2004a;142).

Ideal-type SHI systems have the following components in common (Saltman: 2004b;6–8):

- SHI contributions are independent of health risk or health status.
- Individual contributions are directly tied to income, but usually have a payment ceiling.
- Dependents of SHI contributing members have automatic cover.
- SHI contributions are collected separately from state income taxation. These payments are ring-fenced.
- The organisational structure of SHI systems is pluralistic, involving a wide range of organisational participants. Funds may vary in their membership according to region, religion, or political allegiance, as well as occupational grouping.
- SHI schemes generally provide the same comprehensive benefit package for all members.
- Premiums are collected either directly through a localised sickness insurance fund or a centrally organised fund.
- Members' contributions are distributed to not-for-profit organisations, operated by independent boards, to purchase health care via collective contracts with providers.
- Health care providers can be private, not-for-profit, private for-profit, or public sector.
- All secondary and primary health care providers have contracts with the sickness funds (although they may also provide treatment for those with PHI cover).
- SHI systems generally adopt a 'corporatist' approach,[7] that is, the authority or power of each of the key organisational actors is formally recognised or 'licensed' by the national state.
- Members of sickness funds in principle have a choice about which hospital or doctor they are treated by.

SHI-funded health systems are characterised by a closer interface between the public and private sectors (Blank & Burau:2018;80), although national governments frequently play a key governance role. The state remains the ultimate decision-maker in relation to the range of health and welfare benefits available, the rules for contracting services, determining whether there should be mandatory membership, how contributions are calculated, and the degree of discretion in decision-making enjoyed by sickness funds (Saltman:2004a;5).

SHI schemes face several particular challenges. These include concerns about the long-term financial sustainability and flexibility of these schemes as they rely on contributions from a workforce rather than a tax-paying population. SHI schemes are particularly vulnerable to economic slowdown and a rise in unemployment. Furthermore, schemes rarely raise all the funds necessary and sufficient to meet their statutory responsibilities, as a consequence they are often subsidised by government payments that are generated through direct income taxation. In 2018, these government budget transfers accounted for more than 20% of SHI scheme revenue in 15 out of 28 countries in Europe (WHO Regional Office for Europe:2021;66). Additional monies are also generated by individual co-payments for treatment, as well as so-called 'Sin Taxes' on alcohol and tobacco (Kings Fund:2017).

SHI-funded care is however less cost-effective than health systems funded through direct taxation, reflecting the additional administrative costs incurred by the extra layers of bureaucracy involved. This includes the administration of the schemes themselves, the administration of the regional funds that play an intermediate role in the distribution of health finance and provider contracts, and finally the separate administrative costs of the health care provider organisations. An independent review was commissioned by the British government into potential health funding alternatives to direct taxation two decades ago. The final report concluded that given the evidence available at the time, an alternative SHI funding system for the NHS 'would not deliver a given quality of health care either at a lower cost to the economy or in a more equitable way' (Wanless:2002;para 6.66).

Direct taxation

Within the WHO European Region, 13 countries, including the UK, have some form of direct government taxation as the primary source for UHC funding (WHO Regional Office for Europe:2021;33). Direct taxation funding systems are able to pool the cost of health and financial risk across a whole population to ensure equitable health service coverage. Methods of levying tax vary between countries. In the UK, state revenue for public service spending is raised through general income tax, as well as taxes on consumption, i.e. VAT, and taxes levied on businesses, while in Sweden, for example, public funding for health care comes from both central and local government taxation.

General taxation is an efficient way of raising money given its low administration costs relative to the amount of funding raised (Kings Fund:2017). However, as the burden of health needs increases, so government's are placed in the position of having to make decisions about the proportion of public service spending that should be allocated to health care as against other state commitments. The obvious solution is to raise the levels of general taxation, but this is never popular with the electorate. The dilemma of cutting public services or raising taxes when the economy is experiencing periods of low growth or contraction means that government can be held directly political accountable for whatever choice they finally make. This democratic accountability is largely absent from the SHI funding model.

Hypothecated taxation

Hypothecation is a component of general taxation, usually based on income, levied for a dedicated purpose such as health care. In principle, hypothecation enables transparency, as an individual can see their tax contribution going directly to the health system. Here there is the potential for people to be prepared to pay more (hypothecated) income tax 'if they can see where it is being spent, especially given the strong public support for health care' (Kings Fund:2017). The argument against hypothecation is that the decision-making autonomy of governments to allocate spending budgets according to their own fiscal strategies is undermined by this ring-fencing approach. A final consideration is that because hypothecated taxes are not linked to the requirements of the health system but to the state of the national economy: '(R)ather than determining health spending by how much a tax raises, it should be based on the health needs of the population. Severing this link between need and provision risks wasteful spending when the tax base is buoyant and insufficient budgets when it is depressed' (Doetinchem:2010;5).

Private health insurance (PHI)

In PHI funding schemes, individuals and/or their employers on their behalf, pay insurance contributions into schemes run by for-profit companies. Contributions (or premiums) are based on an individual's health risk that is assessed on the basis of age, family medical history, the existence of pre-existing medical conditions, residence, gender, ethnicity, and a range of other socio-economic factors. Contribution payment levels also vary considerably between different types of PHI scheme, which can provide cover individual's and their families, a whole community, or a group of employees.

PHI is the primary form of health cover in the USA. The majority of Americans acquire insurance cover through their employment, funded by a combination of employee and employer tax-exempt premium contributions. There also exist publicly administered and funded health insurance programmes (usually operated through private insurance companies) such as Medicare for low-income families and Medicare for disabled and older people. Yet nearly 10% of the US population is not enrolled in any private or state health funding scheme. Beyond the USA, some countries fund their health care systems via compulsory or mandatory PHI schemes. There are two countries in Europe who operate this type of funding system, the Netherlands and Switzerland. In Switzerland, health insurance became compulsory for the whole population as recently as 1996. Individuals now pay personal health risk-related premiums to non-profit private insurance companies, while local government plays a role in subsidising the premiums of people with incomes below a specified threshold (WHO Regional Office for Europe:2021;31).

The standard argument presented in favour of PHI funding is that it promotes choice for its users, encourages competition, and drives up standards of care amongst health providers. The argument against is that an unregulated PHI market will engage in 'cherry-picking', excluding individuals with perceived high levels of health risk. This results in significant social inequities as these uninsured population groups have no other choice then to pay for their health care through expensive, non-pooled OOP payments.

PHI premiums are effectively regressive taxes. There is usually no connection between the cost of premiums and personal income levels, so that the cost of insurance is a much higher proportionally for those on lower incomes. PHI schemes incur much greater administrative costs than either direct taxation or SHI 'due to the extra resources required to assess health risk, set premiums, design benefit packages and assess claims' (Kings Fund:2017). Finally, PHI companies are profit-seeking organisations, so that a significant proportion of insurance premium costs are not spent on direct care costs but are paid out as dividends to shareholders.[8]

Supply-side and demand-side strategies for health care 'Cost-Containment'

It was in the mid-1970s, during the first significant post-war global economic recession, that high-income countries with UHC systems first seriously began engage with the potential limits to state health spending. The issue became one of balancing the increasing demand for health and health care costs while facing a substantial reduction in the levels of state revenue due to the dramatic rise in unemployment and loss of profitability. Finding a solution to this fiscal equation applied equally to direct taxation and SHI funding systems. From this policy predicament emerged what became known as 'demand-side' and 'supply-side' cost-containment strategies. Both strategies have been utilised by governments at different times, and sometimes both in tandem. What both these cost-containment strategies have in common is that they are blunt financial instruments.

Demand-side strategies are designed to dampen-down or limit patient health care demands. In PHI-dominated health care systems this process is relatively straightforward. The cost of individual premiums is raised and financial inducements offered to improve the efficiency of health care providers. In SHI-funded systems, OOP payments for services such as a visit to a General Practitioner (GP), or overnight hotel charges in hospitals can be introduced. These additional charges may require that the patient pays the first 100 Euro of any treatment before their social insurance cover becomes available for example, or limiting the reimbursements that are available for certain health services. In direct taxation funded systems such as the UK, co-payment (fixed) charges for prescriptions can and have been raised consistently over the past four decades. While there is evidence that demand-side strategies do reduce system costs in the short term, the consequences of patients delaying essential early treatment because of their reluctance to meet these additional payments, can mean that over the long term, health costs increase.

Supply-side strategies are generally more straightforward to manage in national health care systems as they involve centralised control over expenditure, rather than the complexities associated with de-centralised systems. In SHI-funded systems, supply-side strategies can involve not-for-profit insurance funds reducing their payments to health care providers in order to match their own income generated through employer and employee contributions. In direct taxation systems, government's can cap health care spending much more straightforwardly through national budgeting strategies that balance state spending against revenue over the course of a financial year. But such strategies can also serve to limit capital development (the reduction in programmes of repair and modernisation of hospital buildings is a frequent target for cost-containment), as well slowdown the uptake of new technological innovations that may in the long-term bring about improvements in efficiency and cost-effectiveness. Alternatively, resources can be centrally re-distributed from secondary hospital-based care to primary and preventative care, including strategies such as day surgery centres (Blank et al:2018;107–117).

Concluding comments

In this chapter the importance of analytically separating the trends in health system financing from the discussion of the relative sustainability of the three main types of funding scheme has been emphasised. As the World Health Organisation has noted: '(C)onventional distinctions between SHI and tax-financed schemes are no longer meaningful. These classifications do not determine sources of revenue and they mask the fact that all forms of compulsory prepayment with risk pooling offer people insurance. The key question for policy is how well different health systems do in meeting the universal health coverage (UHC) goals of universal access to health services with financial protection' (WHO Regional Office for Europe:2021;xviii). The WHO concern with global health system sustainability through the achievement of UHC points to the distinct limitations of PHI-funded health care, particularly but not exclusively in medium- and low-income countries. This will be a key focus of concern in the following section of this book.

Notes

1 Detailed descriptions of the health system funding and financing arrangements in low-income countries, specifically Ghana and Kenya are set out in Chapter 6 and in high-income countries, the UK and Germany in Chapter 7.
2 The UN SDG's are discussed in detail in Chapter 5.
3 The OECD defines health spending as the measure of the final consumption of health care goods and services (i.e. current health expenditure) including personal health care (curative care, rehabilitative care, long-term care, ancillary services, and medical goods) and collective services (prevention and public health services as well as health administration), but excluding spending on investments.
4 The analysis of the impact of ageing populations on the demand for health and social care is the primary focus of Chapter 8.
5 Even in contemporary policy analysis, social insurance systems are still referred to as the 'Bismarck model'. The history of social health and welfare insurance in Germany is discussed in Chapter 7.
6 The development of post-war national welfare states is discussed in Chapter 1.
7 Discussed in relation to the German SHI system in Chapter 7.
8 Questions about the sustainability of PHI health funding for health systems in low-income countries are discussed in detail in Chapter 6.

References

Blank, R, Burau, V and Kuhlmann, E (2018) *Comparative Health Policy* (5th Ed). Basingstoke. Palgrave.
Centres for Disease Control and Prevention (2022) Demographic Variation in Health Insurance Coverage: United States 2020. *National Health Statistics Reports.* No 169, February 11, 2022.
Doetinchem, O (2010) *Hypothecation of Tax Revenue for Health.* World Health Report Background Paper, 51. Geneva. WHO.
Freeman, R (2000) *The Politics of Health in Europe Manchester.* Manchester. Manchester University Press.
Kings Fund (2017) *How health care is funded.* www.kingsfund.org.uk (accessed 10/2022).
Kutzen, J, Witter, S, Jowett, M and Bayarsaikhan, D (2017) *Developing a National Health Financing Strategy: A Reference Guide.* Geneva. Switzerland. WHO.
OECD (2022) *Economic Outlook.* www.oecd-ilibrary.org/economics/oecd-economic-outlook_16097408 (accessed 11/2022).
Office of Budget Responsibility (2023) *Economic and Fiscal Outlook – November 2023.* CP 944. www.obr.uk/ (accessed 04/2024).
Saltman, R (2004a) 'Assessing social health insurance systems: present and future policy issues' in Saltman, R, Busse, R, and Figueras, J (eds) *Social Health Insurance Systems in Western Europe.* Maidenhead. Open University Press, pp 141–152.
Saltman, R (2004b) 'Social health insurance in perspective: the challenge of sustained stability' in Saltman, R, Busse, R, and Figueras, J (eds) *Social Health Insurance Systems in Western Europe.* Maidenhead. Open University Press, pp 3–20
Wanless, D (2002) *Securing Our Future Health: Taking a Long-Term View - Final Report.* London. HM Treasury.
World Health Organisation (2022) *Global Expenditure on Health: Rising to the Pandemics Challenges.* Geneva. WHO.
World Health Organisation (2023) *Global Health Expenditure Database.* https://apps.who.int/nha/database/Home/Index/en (accessed 01/2023).
World Health Organisation, Regional Office for Europe (2021) *Spending on Health in Europe – Entering a New Era?* Copenhagen. WHO.

SECTION II
_____

Conceiving and Comparing Health Care Systems

Introduction to Section II

Over two decades ago, the World Health Report published by the WHO noted that:

> (T)oday, health systems in all countries, rich and poor, play a bigger and more influential role in people's lives than ever before. Health systems of some sort have existed for as long as people have tried to protect their health and treat diseases. Traditional practices, often integrated with spiritual counselling and providing both preventive and curative care, have existed for thousands of years and often coexist today with modern medicine. But 100 years ago, organized health systems in the modern sense barely existed. Few people alive then would ever visit a hospital. Most were born into large families and faced an infancy and childhood threatened by a host of potentially fatal diseases ... Infant and child mortality rates were very high, as were maternal mortality rates. Life expectancy was short.
> *(WHO:2000;xiii)*

The WHO report went on to recognise that given their complexity any attempt to provide a universal definition of a health system is necessarily problematic. Nevertheless, the WHO do go on to provide a broad definition: '(T)he resources, actors and institutions related to the financing, regulation and provision of health actions, where health actions are any set of activities whose primary intent is to improve or maintain health' (WHO:2000;7). This definition is consistent with the WHO's founding constitution that stated that health was, 'a state of complete physical, mental and social well-being and not merely the absence of disease or infirmity' (WHO:2020). On this basis, health systems that are designed to maintain the health and well-being of populations should ideally include provision for primary and secondary medical care, but also public health activities that include interventionary disease prevention programmes, health promotion, and other educational activities. A broad-based health system should also promote environmental and climate protection policies, sustainable energy policies, a high standard of housing for all, accessible green spaces in urban settings, workplace well-being, and other activities that can positively shape the social determinants of health in a society.

But recognising that the achievement of 'health for all' necessarily requires collective interventions that go beyond the formal boundaries of health care provision systems, although this is not to dismiss the contribution of clinical medicine in alleviating

DOI: 10.4324/9781003564249-7

physical and mental suffering. It is essential to ensure that the performance of the health care systems we all rely so much upon are performing at the highest possible standards. And, in order to assess the performance of any given health system, it must first be defined as a clear entity (Papinicolis et al:2022). Then it becomes possible to subject to the performance outputs of a given system to the rigours of comparative analysis.

Thirty years ago, health policy analysis was largely focused on the structure and function of the national health care system in which the analyst themselves lived and worked. In part, this insular approach reflected a prevailing and essentially arrogant discourse, which was particularly the case in the UK, that the NHS had nothing to learn from elsewhere in the world. There were also technical limitations also partly explain this narrow analytical focus. Before the construction of digitalised health information systems (HIS), the relative paucity of available analogue data meant that attempting to compare the performance of health systems was a daunting task. But in more recent years, the exponential development of networked HISs and the ready availability of detailed performance output data have opened up new possibilities for comparative health system research. Today, comparative analysis 'offers a virtual test of different policy options, and as such promises evidence-based policy making, policy innovation and, above all, policy success' (Blank et al:2018;274).

The World Bank has stated that comparative analysis is fundamental to being in a position to be able to, 'propose causes of poor health system performance and suggests how reform policies and strengthening strategies can improve performance...(and) contributes to implementation and evaluation' (Berman & Bitran:2011;6). On this basis it is only through comparative assessment that it becomes possible to benchmark areas they are performing above or below expectations within a given health system. Furthermore, comparative system analysis provides these national policymakers, 'with an impetus to understand what is driving reported performance, as well as guidance on where to look for potential solutions' (Papanicolas & Smith:2013;2).

Why is it important to have a global health policy perspective?

This second section of the book is concerned with outlining the methodological issues associated with comparative health systems analysis. A number of dedicated analytical frameworks now exist embracing a wide range of system performance output indicators, and these are explored in the chapters that constitute this second section. However, there is also a concern to provide worked examples of comparative analysis that are not restricted to health systems in high-income countries.

It remains the case that comparative health systems analysis is more commonly undertaken in relation to systems within high-income countries (HICs) than it is between systems in low- and medium-income countries (LICs and MICs). While some of the challenges faced by health systems in LICs specifically relate to the high levels of disease and poverty experienced in many of these countries, the fundamentals of an effective and efficiently performing health system remain fundamentally the same in a wealthy or poor country. One of the probable reasons for the relative paucity of comparative LIC health systems analysis is an ideological one, whether implicit or explicit. This reflects a continuing problematisation of many of these countries as being somehow trapped in a legacy of what has euphemistically been termed 'underdevelopment'.

Over 60 years ago, in a speech concerned with the challenges of implementing progressive social and political reforms in countries characterised by poverty, colonial exploitation, and inequality, The Cuban Revolutionary leader, Che Guevara, raised the issue of nomenclature. This is the process, frequently ideological, of the naming of things and the associated symbolic power that then is attached to these terms. Che argued that behind the apparently uncontroversial use of the term 'underdevelopment' lies a global economic structure that systematically acts in the interests of the richest and most powerful:

> We, politely referred to as "underdeveloped," in truth are colonial, semi-colonial or dependent countries. We are countries whose economies have been distorted by imperialism, which has abnormally developed those branches of industry or agriculture needed to complement its complex economy. "Underdevelopment," or distorted development, brings a dangerous specialization in raw materials, inherent in which is the threat of hunger for all our peoples
>
> *(taken from Historical Exceptions or Vanguard in the Anticolonial Struggle? March 2005; Part 2)*

Colonial-era stereotypes continue to be deployed in labelling sub-Saharan countries as somehow predisposed to failure. This pervading narrative frequently presents Africa as a continent marked by endemic crises, corruption, wars, and ethnic conflict. This uniformly negative presentation of African affairs has become known as 'Afro-pessimism'. This narrative has served to 'justify the continued exploitation of the continent's people and resources by obscuring imperialist practices that undermine the sovereignty of African states (and) ... prevents us from better understanding the challenges or solutions to political problems in post-colonial African countries' (Okath:2023;ix). One of the key objectives of conducting a comparative analysis of the Ghanaian and Kenyan health systems within this book is to contribute, in a modest way, to the breaking-down of some of these misrepresentations and distortions.

Following the comparative analysis of these two African nations, a more established comparison, that between the UK and German health care systems is undertaken. The history of collective forms of health care provision in both countries date back to the end of the nineteenth century, when it became apparent that only the national state as a 'collective actor' could provide the infrastructure that was required to sustain these increasingly complex national economies. Following the trauma of the Second World War in both countries, the demands of post-war economic reconstruction and political renewal led onto the construction new institutions of health and welfare predicated on the principles of universalism and equity to meet the social and health needs of their respective populations. Today, both health systems face the challenge of ageing populations and the financial constraints associated with an era of economic globalisation.

References

Berman, P and Bitran, R (2011) *Health Systems Analysis for Better Health System Strengthening.* Washington, DC. The World Bank.

Blank, R, Burau, V and Kuhlmann, E (2018) *Comparative Health Policy* (5th Ed). Basingstoke. Palgrave.

March, I (2005) *The Che Reader: Writings on Politics and Revolution.* www.oceanbooks.com.

Okath, KO (2023) *Red Africa: Reclaiming Revolutionary Black Politics*. London. Verso Books.

Papanicolas, I and Smith, P (2013) 'Introduction' in Papanicolas, I and Smith, P (eds) *Health System Performance Comparison: An Agenda for Policy, Information and Research*. Maidenhead. Open University Press, pp 1–28.

Papanicolas, I, Rajan, D, Karanikolos, M and Figueras, J (2022) 'Assessing health systems performance for universal health coverage: rationale and approach' in Papanicolas, I, Rajan, D, Karanikolas, M, Soucat, A, and Figueras, J (eds) *Health System Performance Assessment: A Framework for Policy Analysis*. Brussels. Observatory on Health Systems and Policy/WHO, pp 1–7.

World Health Organisation (2000) *World Health Report 2000: Health Systems – Improving Performance*. Geneva. Switzerland. World Health Organization.

World Health Organisation (2020) *Basic Documents: 49th Edition*. https://apps.who.int/gb/bd/pdf_files/BD_49th-en.pdf (accessed 10/2022).

CHAPTER 5

Comparing and evaluating health system outcomes

A taxonomy of comparative health system evaluation

Four decades ago, if the comparative analyses of health systems occurred at all, it was generally of the 'snapshot' variety, resting on a single metric, total health care expenditure (THE) measured as a proportion of Gross Domestic Product (GDP[1]). The limitations of relying on this comparator was that alone it could not account for differences in the structure, provision, quality, equity, and overall performance of health care systems. Today, comparative analyses draw on a much broader range of quantitative as well as qualitative indicators. It also follows that there is no one universally agreed methodological approach to comparative systems research, nor can there be given the range of theoretical differences and purposes for which comparative health systems evaluative research is undertaken.

Marmor and Wendt's (2012) taxonomy set out in Table 5.1 identifies four main foci of comparative health system research differentiated by their position on two analytical axes. The first axis distinguishes between research that is orientated towards health care institutions and policy actors and those that focus on the organisational structure of systems. The second axis distinguishes between comparative studies that are process-orientated and those that focus on measurable system output differences. However, the authors are at pains to point out that their taxonomy is constituted by ideal typologies and that in practice there are interactions between these analytical dimensions (Marmor & Wendt:2012;18).

Central to this taxonomy is the implicit understanding that health care organisations are not closed systems. The measurement of comparative system functionality and efficiency may be utilised to assess the performance of any given health system, but these outcomes also reflect the specific social and economic context in which the system operates. Distinct historical and institutional contexts produce very specific combinations of health policy actors. As Wendt has more recently noted, this contextual variance can result in: '(D)ifferent consequences for health reform processes, for the coordination of health care systems with other fields of social policy, for the level and quality of health care provision and the financial burden for those in need, and for health and health inequalities' (Wendt:2022;54).

Output-orientated comparative systems research has expanded in recent years, this has been facilitated by the development of national networked health information systems (HIS) able to collect an array of performance data. This data is collated within large open access databases hosted for example by the OECD (2021), the WHO (2023a), and

Table 5.1 Dimensions of comparative health system analysis

Form of Analysis	Health Policy Actors & Institutions	Organisational Structure of Health Care Systems
Process Orientated	(a) Roles of political institutions and policy-actors in framing health policy	(c) Funding, regulation, and governance mechanisms constituting organisational structures
Outcome Orientated	(b) Values and ideologies, both implicit and explicit, shaping the governance of health policy reform and development	(d) Measurable Indicators of system performance such as access, equity, quality of care, patient satisfaction, etc.

Source: Adapted from Marmor and Wendt (2012).

the European Observatory on Health Systems and Policies. However, process-orientated comparative research that examines organisational functionality at the level of governance, funding, policymaking, and goal-setting also continues to occupy a pivotal role in comparative systems analysis. Wendt's (2009) analytical framework that is outlined in Table 5.3 is very much process-orientated and this is because its specific purpose is to 'unfold the institutional structures of developed health care systems' (Wendt:2022;57).

Comparative performance ranking indexes: purposes and limitations

The contemporary version of the 'snapshot' comparison of health systems are ranking indexes. These indexes produce 'scores' for the performance of a limited range of health systems, usually only in HIC's only, and explicitly not intended to be systematic comparative analyses. They generally employ a variety of generalised performance measures, with a deal of 'confusion and debate over which indicators to use, what statistical weighting to place on each, and how to present the information in ranked format' (Schütte et al:2018;2). As a consequence, the different ranking indexes can often produce quite different scores for the same country. Three of the better-known ranking indexes are outlined below, and attention is drawn to their general purpose's and to their limitations.

The Euro Health Consumer Index was published annually from 2005 to 2018 and claimed to measure the 'consumer friendliness' of 36 European health care systems (not all of which were EU member states). It drew on just three indices of health system performance: patient rights, waiting times for treatment, and range of services provided to patients. As the name implied, this was a consumer index of health care services but was not commercially sponsored. In 2017, the Netherlands achieved the highest overall score on the index with the UK being ranked 15th (EHCI:2017). Quite how European health care consumers were supposed to utilise these findings was never explained, certainly the option of crossing borders to receive the best care (based only on these three indicators) was a non-starter. In 2018, the index ceased to be produced, and it was not a coincidence that this followed criticism from both academic and clinical sources. The over-arching critique was that the consumer index was based on arbitrary cut-off points, with no obvious logic to the maximum scores allocated to different indicators and that it utilised a mix of trends over time as well as cross-sectional rankings (Cylus et al:2016).

The Bloomberg global business information network is responsible for the annual production of an eponymous health index. This particular 'efficiency' ranking index seeks to identify the 'best and worst' health systems, but again utilises just three weighted metrics: life expectancy, health care costs per capita, and costs as a percentage of GDP. These metrics are applied to publicly available data for 57 HICs (drawn largely from the World Bank and International Monetary Fund), all of which have populations of at least 5 million, GDP per capita of at least $5,000, and life expectancy of at least 70 years. A health care efficiency score is produced for each country. The Bloomberg index for 2020 that included an adjustment for the relative impact of COVID-19 placed Singapore in the No. 1 spot as the 'most efficient' and the US Health Care System as the least 'efficient' of these HICs. Yet as Bloomberg themselves acknowledge, they are not a dedicated health research organisation: '(Our) Best (and Worst) rankings seek to enlighten and entertain readers on topical issues of immediate and perennial interest in business, economics, investing, lifestyle, personal finance and politics & policy' (Bloomberg:2023).

A third example has been that produced on a periodic basis by the Washington-based Commonwealth Fund, a US private research foundation since 2004. This ranking system utilises five 'domains' ('access to care', 'care process', 'administrative efficiency', 'equity', and 'health care outcomes'), which are assessed by a total of 71 separate measures in order to compare the performance of 11 high-income health systems (The Commonwealth Fund:2023). The Commonwealth Fund reports draw on specially commissioned international surveys of patients and primary care physicians' experiences, combined with standardised Organisation for Economic Co-operation and Development (OECD) and World Health Organisation (WHO) system performance data. A 'normalised' score for each health system is then produced and calculated as the difference between the specific scores for a given country and the mean of the other 10 countries, divided by the standard deviation of the results for each measure (Schneider et al:2021;17). The stated goal of this ranking index is to provide: 'International comparisons to allow the public, policymakers, and health care leaders to see alternative approaches to delivering health care, ones that might be borrowed to build better health systems that yield better health outcomes' (Schneider et al:2021;14). The most recent Commonwealth Funding ranking was published in 2021 and placed Norway in the top position and the US health system at the bottom.

The Commonwealth Fund ranking system is more comprehensive than the two ranking indexes previously discussed. It acknowledges its own limitations which relate to the fact that while the detailed patients and physicians survey data is rich in detail, it does not 'capture important dimensions that might be obtained from medical records or administrative data' (Schneider et al:2021;18). The Commonwealth Fund reports provide no details of the statistical weighting used in relation to the relative contribution of each of its five domains. Finally, in attempting to find common denominators of performance across 11 diverse health systems, inevitably there will be a lack of contextual specificity. Comparing countries with similar levels of per capita income and wealth does not mean that the index is sensitive to the social, economic, and political context in which these health systems operate. The unique characteristics of health care provision within individual countries can disappear when reliance is placed on large-scale cross-national data sets. Finally, seemingly similar nomenclature used to describe aspects of health care provision does not always describe precisely the same constituents across systems. Without sensitivity to these cultural differences there is a potential for false or misinformed assumptions to be drawn when comparing systems.

Output-orientated comparative analysis

The objective of output-orientated analysis is to provide a comprehensive range of 'performance' metrics that can be drawn upon in the comparison of two or more health care systems. In this section, two output-orientated assessment frameworks are presented. The first example (see Table 5.2) draws in part, on the methodology adopted by the WHO within its 'health system strengthening' strategy (WHO:2000). The second framework (see Table 5.3) has been specifically designed to compare high-income European health care systems characterised by universal health coverage (UHC).

The World Health Report was intended as an assessment framework for national health policymakers, 'as they need to know why health systems perform in certain ways and what they can do to improve the situation' (WHO:2000;xii). The self-assured tone that was adopted within the report seeks to explain why and how national health policy-makers should seek to adopt the principles that inform the WHO health system assessment framework. If they do so, then health resources are to be directed to the improvement of health system performance for the greatest population 'heath gain'.

Table 5.2 A framework for comparative health system analysis: as applied to low-income developing countries

System Evaluative Categories	Indicators
(1) Quality & Effectiveness	■ Health service availability and readiness ■ Meeting international disease management standards and regulations ■ Implementation of patient safety and quality assurance standards
(2) Patient & Population Outcomes	■ Information systems: Monitoring, evaluation, and timely dissemination of reliable data ■ Population coverage of public health programmes ■ Social differences in morbidity & mortality rates
(3) Equity & Financial Sustainability	■ Distributive Justice: How are the benefits and costs of health care distributed? ■ Health System Financing: Cost-risk sharing and the role of public and private Insurance funding
(4) Governance & Accountability	■ Health system capacity for reform and quality improvement ■ Implementation and enforcement of regulatory frameworks across all system activities
(5) Efficiency	■ Allocative efficiency of health system ■ Technical efficiency of health system
(6) Access & Responsiveness	■ Accessibility of health services ■ Integrated health care services: Example - Integrated Management Childhood Illness (IMCI) ■ User experiences

Source: Adapted from Basu et al (2012); WHO (2000, 2007); WHO AFRO (2022).

The pathway to progress is seen, 'to depend crucially on how well systems carry out four vital functions: service provision, resource generation, financing, and stewardship' (WHO:2000;xi). The World Health Report is concerned to establish the core principles for the achievement of equitable and sustainable health systems, but it is much less specific on policy practicalities.

Seven years on, and belatedly recognising the limitations of the original World Health Report, the WHO published *Everybody's Business – Strengthening Health Systems to Improve Outcomes: WHO's Framework for Action* (WHO:2007). The subtitle of this document indicates the change of focus and sets out a more direct advisory role for the WHO in building the capacity of member states not only in health policy development but also in relation to organisational governance and institutional management. The emphasis of the 2000 report had been the interdependence of the four identified system functions, the 2007 document recognised that many health systems, particularly those in low-income developing countries (LIDCs) as well as medium-income countries (MICs), required support to overcome what were described as 'ineffectively integrated' health services (WHO:2007;8). To this end, the 2007 document sets out an integrated framework composed of six ideal-type system 'building blocks', each with an accompanying set of detailed priorities. These building blocks are (i) Service delivery. (ii) Health workforce. (iii) Health Information. (iv) Medical products, vaccines, and technologies. (v) Financing. (vi) Leadership and governance. The stated intention of the WHO in developing this ideal-type framework was, 'as the basis for dialogue with partners, to inform internal staff development and learning, or as an input into operational planning at all levels' (WHO:2007;35).

The six building blocks were never designed nor intended to constitute an assessment tool for comparative systems analysis. So it for this reason that while the six evaluative categories set out in Table 5.2 are informed by the WHO building blocks they are not coterminous with them. They are specifically designed to assess the challenges faced by, as well as the performance outputs of, health care systems found in LIDCs. These evaluative categories also include performance indicators that derive from two other sources. One is a widely cited study[2] concerned with the relative effectiveness of the private and public health care sectors in a range of LIDCs (Basu et al:2012). The other source is the 'Health Situation Analysis' that forms a key assessment tool in the WHO African Region *Atlas of Health Statistics* (WHO AFRO:2022). The methodological assumptions that underpin each of these six evaluative categories and their descriptors are outlined below.[3]

Quality

Although it is a relatively arbitrary concept, 'quality' is nevertheless widely utilised as the basis for assessing health service outputs and performance. A key consideration must therefore be to ensure the robustness of the indicators that are used to measure 'quality'. One approach is to equate 'quality' with service capacity levels, standing as a macro-measure of the range of provision in a given system. A second use is as a micro-evaluation of individual patient experiences of service delivery, where it is essentially a measure of perceived 'value'. A third contextual use of 'quality' is in relation to clinical effectiveness. The latter is generally defined as the use of evidence-based approaches in determining the most clinically optimal course of treatment for a patient. Each of these interpretations of 'quality' may be a precondition of the others, but this does not mean they are necessarily congruent one with the other. The lack of specificity in the use of 'quality' in relation to system performance is a trait that unfortunately continues to occur in the more descriptive health service evaluation literature.

Patient and population outcomes

The use of population or patient outcomes is a relatively crude indicator of health system performance that serves to marginalise the complexity of the social and environmental interactions that contribute to these outcomes. Nevertheless, mortality and morbidity trend data, standing in as a proxy measure, continues to be the default approach to measuring patient and population outcomes. It is only at a highly reductive level that mortality and morbidity statistics can be considered to indicate the relative effectiveness of health interventions, whether that is through public health programmes or timely access to health care services.

Equity and sustainability

The WHO defines equity as: '(T)he absence of unfair, avoidable or remediable differences among groups of people, whether those groups are defined socially, economically, demographically, or geographically or by other dimensions of inequality (e.g. sex, gender, ethnicity, disability, or sexual orientation) …. *Health equity is achieved when everyone can attain their full potential for health and well-being*' (WHO:2023b – emphasis in original). This definition explicitly links to the popular idea of 'fairness', but it is also very close to the ethical principle of 'distributive justice'. Applying the concept of equity as an evaluative output category generally focuses on whether the risks, costs, and benefits of health care are shared proportionally within a health system. This particular application also embraces the idea that health care is a 'special' case and that it should be treated differently from other goods and services that are distributed and consumed unequally within societies (Daniels:1983;2).

Sustainable development in relation to the performance of a health care system is generally linked to the optimisation of resources. Sustainable, not only in terms of environmental responsibility, but also in relation to the prudential management of finance and funding, as well as the use of the human resources central to the effective functioning of any health system. Yet specifying measurable indices of a 'sustainable' health system remains a complex matter. One influential approach is that adopted by the UN/WHO in the construction of their 17 Sustainable Development Goals or SDGs (WHO:2015). These goals represent ideal-type social and economic objectives that are explicitly intended to be applicable to all countries, not just so-called 'developing' countries. Specifically in terms of the sustainability of health systems, the relevant SDG states that: 'A comprehensive health system (is one that) provides complete coverage with fully-staffed and well-managed health services, protecting users from financial risk' (WHO:2015).

Governance

Governance is a multi-layered and dynamic concept, but essentially it is used as a heuristic or schematic to stress the relational or *process* aspects of decision-making power and authority.[4] Governance as a health system evaluative category focuses on the assessment of public accountability and resource allocation transparency, as well as the existence of regulatory mechanisms governing professional practice and patient safety.

Efficiency

This concept is most frequently associated with the optimisation of resources in health care systems. Health economists generally disaggregate this concept into the following three separate but linked forms for analytical convenience (a) 'Technical efficiency' referring to the optimal use of system resources in the delivery or production of a given health intervention. Crudely put, this equates to the least possible resource input for the best possible output. (b) 'Cost-effectiveness' referring to the process of assessing the costs and outcomes of alternative options for health policy interventions; this can also include maintaining the current status quo. It is generally calculated as a formulaic ratio. One example would be the attempt to measure the quality of life of an individual or of a cohort of patients assessed as 'life year's gained', balanced against the cost of a given health resource or clinical intervention.[5] A critique of this approach is that, 'cost-effectiveness thresholds are commonly mistaken for affordability thresholds' (Guindo:2012;11). (c) 'Allocative efficiency' refers to the distribution of resources across an entire sector of health care interventions. The objective being to achieve the maximum possible socially desired outcome for the available resources (Hutubessey et al:2003).

Disaggregating the concept of efficiency has a clear practical utility, but there is a further analytical hurdle to clear, and this relates to the complexity and sheer scale of attempting an efficiency evaluation of a whole health system. It is for this reason that system efficiency assessment necessarily requires analysing performance at different operational levels of a system. At the *micro-level* of the individual patient, the focus would be on assessing the efficiency of provider care. Here an important consideration is that evidence from practice indicates that: 'a high level of efficiency cannot be achieved without reducing quality or clinical effectiveness of healthcare service provision due to the potential trade off between them' (lo Storto & Goncharuk:2017). At the *meso-level* of organisational structuring, the focus would be relative efficiency in the use of provider resources. This may, for example concern the relative balance of health resources directed at primary preventative family and community-based care, as against secondary hospital-based individual treatment. On this point, attention has been drawn to situations where focusing solely on technical efficiency without regard to allocative efficiency 'means you could just end up doing more and more of activities that contribute little to health' (HEU:2022). At the *macro-level* of the health system, efficiency might be evaluated in terms of the proportion of national resources utilised in maintaining structures of health care intervention, as against resources directed towards improvements in population living standards.

Access

Access is generally conceived as the interface between service users and health care resources. By convention, it is evaluated as a function of the balance between health care service supply and demand factors. On this basis, health care access is not purely a question of being able to consult a health professional for advice, further referral, or for medical treatment. Access can also represent the extent to which health needs may be only partially met due to the limited availability of health resources. Alternate approaches to evaluating access include assessment of patient or user experiences, the physical accessibility of health care facilities, as well as the geographic proximity to, and the availability of transport links to clinics and hospitals for local communities.

However, widening 'access' is not always compatible with the goal of universalism. The principle of universalism generally assumes a minimum, but not maximum, level of care for individuals in need. Generally speaking health systems cannot 'sustain unlimited amounts of resources for the few' (Blank et al:2018;116).

****

Conducting a comparative assessment of the output performance of health systems in HICs is fundamentally the same process as in LIDCs. Nevertheless, there are also important differences between those countries where health systems constitute an integral component of universal welfare state provision, such as in the UK and Germany, and health systems in LIDCs (as well as MICs) where universal health coverage is very much the exception.

Claus Wendt of the Mannheim Centre for European Social Research (MZES) developed a framework[6] for comparative system analysis that sought to take account of universal provision that is a characteristic of health care provision in the majority of European countries. As Wendt notes, 'comparisons that rely on broad organizational and financial principles are not sufficient for gaining a better understanding of healthcare systems. Since healthcare systems serve to provide care for those in need, comparisons first and foremost have to concentrate on healthcare provision as well as on how access to health service providers is regulated' (Wendt:2009;432). This characteristic output-orientated framework includes seven evaluative categories, with each category having an associated set of indicators; together these are set out in Table 5.3.

The rationale underpinning Wendt's evaluative categories will be discussed below under four general headings: (a) Total Expenditure. (b) Funding Systems. (c) Health Care Provision. (d) Specific Institutional characteristics.[7]

Total health care expenditure (THE)

THE is the sum of all health care spending in a given country. This includes both outpatient and inpatient care within both the public and the private health care sectors, public health activities linked to disease prevention, as well as social care for people living with chronic illness and disability. In terms of social care, this spending is included under the THE heading only if these services are provided by the health care system itself, but not if provided under the auspices of local or regional government (as is the case of England and Wales). THE is generally represented as a percentage of Gross Domestic or National Product (GDP or GNP), or sometimes as a per capita monetary amount (the average cost of health care spending per individual member of the population). It should be noted that THE is only weakly correlated to the numbers of health care staff employed within a given health care system. This usually reflects national differences in staffing costs.

Health care financing

As Wendt has noted, '(I)n some comparative studies, the mode of financing[8] is taken to be the main or even sole indicator for classifying health care systems' (2009;434). Within Wendt's own framework, funding as an evaluative category is assessed on the basis of the relative mix of public and private funding within the overall system. Generally the lower the proportional funding contribution of the state, then the

Table 5.3 Evaluative categories for comparative health system analysis: as applied to European welfare state systems

System Evaluative Categories	Indicators
(1) Health Care Expenditure	Total Health expenditure (THE) – Represented as a percentage of GDP, or sometimes as a per capita amount.
(2) Health Care Funding Mix	Public-Private Mix of Financing – The level of state guarantee of access to health care
(3) 'Privatisation of Risk'	Share of health care costs in a system individually covered through private insurance schemes and OOP.
(4) Health Service Provision	Service density; Health care staff to population ratios; The balance of primary and secondary care provision; Waiting times for treatment; etc.
(5) Entitlement to Health care	On the basis of: Citizenship; Compulsory Social insurance, or Private insurance contributions?
(6) Remuneration of health professions	Doctors payment per capita basis, 'fee-for service', or salary – Indicator of the degree of relative autonomy of health care professionals
(7) Patient's Access to Service Providers	The degree to which patients' access to health care is regulated – free choice or gate-keeping system, or whether referral requires additional payments.

Source: Adapted from Wendt (2009).

higher the proportion of costs borne by individuals, either through private insurance schemes or additional out-of-pocket (OOP) payments. This ratio is assumed to indicate the relative inequality of access to health care and so is termed the 'privatisation of (health) risk'.

Health care provision

Health Care Provision, in the language of health economics, constitutes the 'supply side' of a health care system. Health care is a particularly labour intensive activity, and as such employee costs represent a high proportion of the overall expenditure of a health system (typically over 70% in EU countries). Indicators of the 'supply' side of provision would include the 'density ratio' of numbers of health care professionals, as well as numbers of hospital beds vis-à-vis the population as a whole. Rather more precise indicators of health care provision include (i) The ratio of sickness benefit payouts to earnings replacement. (ii) Health care coverage ratios – formally 100% in countries with universal coverage provision. (iii) Waiting times for treatment measured in days. (iv) The length of the payment contribution period required for access to treatment – this is particularly relevant to health systems characterised by high levels of PHI funding. Further indices of health care provision would include the relative emphasis placed within a system on primary health care provision, for example, the number of General Practitioners' (GPs), community nurses, and pharmacists per head of population, as against secondary care provision (in-patient hospital facilities) in a given system (Wendt:2009;435). The former is generally indicative of a greater emphasis placed on disease prevention generally seen to be a more cost-effective use of health resources. However, there also needs to be sufficient levels of secondary care provision to manage health emergencies and high levels of chronic disease in a population, not to mention the unknown requirements for beds during an epidemic or pandemic, COVID-19 being an apt example.

Specific institutional characteristics

■ *Entitlement to health care*: This evaluative category includes an assessment of health care system accessibility (discussed above), this in turn reflects the individual entitlement features of any given health care system. Entitlement can be a right of citizenship or of a proven health need. Entitlement is also directly linked to individual monetary contributions, this is especially the case in PHI-based systems, and to a lesser extent in SHI-based systems. Entitlement to health care provision in the UK is based on a right of residence, not citizenship nor taxation payments, but some forms of treatment do require additional OOP payments such as dental care.

■ *Remuneration received by doctors*: This evaluative category can include payments to doctors based on fee-for-service, per case, or per capita (the number of patients on a surgery's list, as found in the UK), or by payment of a salary. There is evidence that the form of reimbursement influences how medical professionals manage their workload, it also is an indication of the relative autonomy of doctors within a particular health system. For example in the UK, NHS doctors are employees of secondary care provider organisations, whereas the majority of GPs are independent contractors).

■ *Patients access to service providers*: This institutional characteristic assessed as an evaluative category focuses on whether a particular health system enables individual patients to have a free choice of doctors (self-referral), or if they are required to register with a GP, who then acts as the 'gatekeeper' for further referral to more specialist health care. A further factor that has to be assessed is whether a referral incurs further payments for individual patients.

Conclusion

An output-orientated analytical framework for comparing the performance of health systems should ideally be able to link its constitutive evaluative categories together in order to produce an overall assessment of system functionality. Comparative assessment frameworks should also be able to identify inconsistencies or 'gaps' between the formal objectives (health policy), and the actual health care outputs in a given system. Frameworks that utilise a relatively limited palate of indicators, such as the country ranking indexes that are described above, tell us little about the context nor functionality of a given health system as it is experienced by the populations in those countries.

Notes

1 GDP is the standard measure of the value added created through the production of goods and services in a country during a certain period. As such, it also measures the income earned from that production, or the total amount spent on final goods and services – less imports (OECD:2023).

2 As of January 2024, Basu et al's (2012) paper has been cited nearly 1000 time, according to Google Scholar.

3 The evaluative categories presented in Table 5.2 are utilised in the comparative assessment of the Ghanaian and Kenyan health systems that is set out in Chapter 6.

4 The concept of governance in the context of the management of health organisations was discussed in detail in Chapter 3.

5 Cost-effectiveness assessed by means of the formulaic QALYS (quality adjusted life years) is the approach adopted by the National Institute for Health and Care excellence (NICE) in the UK.

6 As of January 2024, Wendt's (2009) paper has been cited in other academic papers and reports over 370 times, according to Google Scholar.

7 The evaluative categories in Table 5.3 are utilised in the comparative assessment of the German and UK health systems as set out in Chapter 7.

8 Wendt does have a tendency to conflate the terms 'financing' and 'funding' in relation to health care provision in his evaluative framework. The issue with the lack of specificity when using the both terms is the focus of discussion in Chapter 4.

References

Basu, S, Andrews, J, Kishore, S, Panjabi, R and Stuckler, D (2012) Comparative performance of private and public healthcare systems in low- and middle-income countries: a systematic review, *Public Library of Science (PLoS) Medicine*, vol. 9, no. 6, 1–13.

Blank, R, Burau, V and Kuhlmann, E (2018) *Comparative Health Policy* (5th Ed). Basingstoke. Palgrave.

Bloomberg UK (2023) *Bloomberg Best (and Worst)*. https://www.bloomberg.com/graphics/best-and-worst/ (accessed 12/2023).

Commonwealth Fund (2023) *Tools and Data Resources*. https://www.commonwealthfund.org/series/mirror-mirror-comparing-health-systems-across-countries (accessed 12/2023).

Cylus, J, Nolte, E, Figueras, M and McKee, M (2016) What, if anything, does the euro health consumer index actually tell us? *British Medical Journal Blogs*, February 9th, 2016.

Daniels, N (1983) 'Health care needs and distributive justice' in Bayer, R, Caplan, A and Daniels, N (eds) *In Search of Equity: Health Needs and Health Care System*. New York. Springer Press, pp 1–41

Euro Health Consumer index (2017) https://healthpowerhouse.com/media/EHCI-2017/EHCI-2017-report.pdf (accessed 04/18).

Guindo, L, Wagner, M, Baltussen, R, Rindress, D, Van til, J, Kind, P and Goetghebeur, M (2012) From efficacy to equity: literature review of decision criteria for resource allocation and healthcare decision making, *Cost Effectiveness and Resource Allocation*, vol. 10, no. 9, 1–13.

Health Economic Unit (2022) *Allocative Efficiency*. https://healtheconomicsunit.nhs.uk (accessed 12/2023).

Hutubessy, R, Chisholm, D and Edejer, T (2003) Generalized cost-effectiveness analysis for national-level priority-setting in the health sector, *Cost Effective Resource Allocation*, vol. 1, no. 1, 1–8.

lo Storto, C and Goncharuk, C (2017) Efficiency vs effectiveness: a benchmarking study on European healthcare systems, *Economics and Sociology*, vol. 10, no. 3, 102–115.

Marmor, T and Wendt, C (2012) Conceptual frameworks for comparing healthcare politics and policy, *Health Policy*, vol. 107, 11–20.

OECD (2021) *Health at a Glance*. https://doi.org/10.1787/ae3016b9-en (accessed 10/2022).

OECD (2023) *OECD National Accounts Statistics*. https://doi.org/10.1787/na-data-en (accessed 07/2023).

Schneider, E, Shah, A, Doty, M, Tikkanen, R, Fields, K and Williams, R (2021) *Mirror, Mirror 2021*. Washington, DC. The Commonwealth Fund. August 2021.

Schütte, S, Marin Acevedo, P and Flahault, A (2018) Health systems around the world: a comparison of existing health system rankings, *Journal of Global Health*, vol. 8, no. 1, 1–9.

Wendt, C (2009) Mapping European healthcare systems: a comparative analysis, *Journal of European Social Policy*, vol. 19, no. 5, 432–445.

Wendt, C (2022) 'Comparative research on health and health care' in Nelson, K, Nieuwenhuis, R and Yerkes, M (eds) *Social Policy in Changing European Societies: Research Agendas for the 21st Century*. Cheltenham. Edward Elgar Publishing, pp 50–65.

World Health Organisation (2000) *World Health Report 2000: Health Systems – Improving Performance*. Geneva. World Health Organization.

World Health Organisation (2007) *Everybody's Business: Strengthening Health Systems to Improve Health Outcomes.* Geneva, Switzerland. WHO.

World Health Organisation (2015) *Sustainable Development Goals.* www.who.int (accessed 10/2022).

World Health Organisation (2023a) *Global Health Expenditure Database.* https://apps.who.int/nha/database/Home/Index/en (accessed 01/2023).

World Health Organisation (2023b) *Health Topics – Health Equity.* https://www.who.int (accessed 10/2023).

World Health Organisation, Regional Office for Africa (2022) *Atlas of African Health Statistics.* https://aho.afro.who.int/publications (accessed 08/2023).

CHAPTER 6

Ghana and Kenya

A comparative analysis of health systems in low-income developing countries

The nomenclature of economic and social development

If you have recently read a newspaper article or academic paper that discusses the 'uneven' impact of some aspect of globalisation, whether that is economic, political, social, or climate change, then you are likely to have encountered the variety of terminology that are used to differentiate clusters of countries.

In the 1950s and 1960s, the differentiation of countries was predicated on the politics of the 'cold war'. The USA and other Western Powers who were members of NATO (North Atlantic Treaty Organisation) tied into a military self-defence pact were self-defined as 'First World'. Those countries that self-identified as communist regimes and signatories of the Warsaw Pact were labelled 'Second World'. While the rest of the world, which disproportionately consisted of economically marginalised countries, many of which were former imperial colonies, were designated as the 'Third World'. The latter term soon took on the status of a catch-all stereotype.

In the 1970s, global institutions such as the United Nations, the World Bank, and the WHO began to draw on the phraseology of 'development' in order to describe the relative economic status of countries. The term 'development' was primarily used in the reductionist sense of defining countries only in terms of their relative (that is to Western countries) economic performance. But there was often also a sub-text in play where the term 'development' was used by former colonial powers to infer a form of cultural inferiority, and it was only in the late 1990s that this attitude finally beginning to change. In 1997, the United Nations adopted Resolution 51/240 also known as the 'Agenda for Development'. This resolution defined 'development' in its very first paragraph, in essentially tautological terms, as follows: 'Development is a multidimensional undertaking to achieve a higher quality of life for all people. Economic development, social development and environmental protection are interdependent and mutually reinforcing components of sustainable development. Sustained economic growth is essential to the economic and social development of all countries. In particular developing countries' (UN:1997;1–2).

Today, the United Nations routinely classifies all countries into one of three categories of development; 'developed economies; economies in transition; and developing economies' (UN:2022). In order to designate the relevant level of 'development'

DOI: 10.4324/9781003564249-9

of a country, the UN also utilises a metric termed the 'Human Development Index' (HDI) (UNDP:2023a). The HDI considers a broad range of factors, including economic growth, life expectancy, health, education, and quality of life. The highest possible HDI score is a 1.0, and any country that scores less than .80 is considered to be 'developing'. In 2021, The United Nations Development Programme (UNDP) HDI gave Ghana a score of 0.632 (in the HDI 'high' tier) and Kenya a score of 0.575 (in the HDI 'medium' tier).

To further add to this nomenclature of 'development', the UN also draws on the World Bank classificatory system that categorises countries by per capita gross national income (GNI), divided into high-income, upper-middle income, lower-middle income or low income bands. The threshold levels of GNI per capita are those established by the World Bank. Currently a 'low income' country is classified as having a GNI of less than $1,046 (World Bank:2022). Still further classificatory layers are also utilised by the UN and its associated institutions. Since 1971, the UN has identified a large group of countries as marked by, 'severe structural impediments to sustainable development … (which) are highly vulnerable to economic and environmental shocks and have low levels of human assets'[1] (UN:2021). These countries are classified as 'Least Developed Countries' or LDCs, there are currently 46 LDC's, 33 of which are on the African continent (UN:2022).

The application of nomenclature is never neutral, and the countries so classified do not always accept their imposed 'label'. For example, in 2021 the Ghanaian Ministry of Finance issued a press release taking exception to the International Monetary Fund (IMF) classifying Ghana as a 'low income country'. The press release ended by stating that: 'We wish to reassure all Ghanaians that Ghana is still classified as a Lower-Middle Income Country' or LIDC (Republic of Ghana MoF:2021). LMIC is indeed how the World Bank classifies Ghana, but this only takes account of per capita income (as described above). The IMF does not actually classify Ghana as 'low income country', but as one of 59 countries that it designates as 'low income developing countries' (LIDC). LIDCs contain one-fifth of the global population but only account for 4% of global output (IMF:2019). LIDC is essentially a portmanteau, one that combines the UN's 'developing countries' classification, with the 'low income' classification utilised by global financial institutions. Throughout this chapter, in order to ensure some level of nomenclature consistency, both Ghana and Kenya will be labelled as 'LIDC'. This how both Kenya and Ghana are most frequently, although not exclusively, classified in the comparative health policy literature.

Sustainable development goals (SDGs) and the achievement of universal health coverage (UHC)

The purpose of this section is to outline the prominent role played by two key and long-standing global institutions, the World Health Organisation and the United Nations, in the promotion of sustainable health system development. Both of these institutions have been proactive in developing ideal-type frameworks that have set the standards for the promotion of greater efficiency in the use of resources in the delivery of health care. In September 2015, the Heads of State and Government and High Representatives met at the United Nations Headquarters in New York to adopt 17 Sustainable Development

Goals (SDGs). The formal declaration that was issued following this meeting contains the following summary statement:

> On behalf of the peoples we serve, we have adopted a historic decision on a comprehensive, far-reaching and people-centred set of universal and transformative Goals and targets. We commit ourselves to working tirelessly for the full implementation of this Agenda by 2030. We recognize that eradicating poverty in all its forms and dimensions, including extreme poverty, is the greatest global challenge and an indispensable requirement for sustainable development. We are committed to achieving sustainable development in its three dimensions – economic, social and environmental – in a balanced and integrated manner. We will also build upon the achievements of the Millennium Development Goals and seek to address their unfinished business
>
> *(UN:2015)*

It is the expectation of the United Nations that the achievement of all 17 of the SDGs will directly contribute to the improvement in the health and living standards of populations. SDG3 ('Good health and well-being') specifically focuses on a country's health policy and how this can best be directed towards ensuring healthy lives and promoting well-being for all ages. Making progress on SDG3, as well as SDG10 ('Reduced inequalities'), combined with progress on all the other 15 sustainability goals, is explicitly linked to the achievement of universal health coverage (UHC) in UN member states.

UHC is a multi-dimensional concept, but it is generally operationalised as an institutionalised and layered framework of rights guaranteed by a national state. Firstly, as a legal framework requiring national governments to provide health care services to all irrespective of income or status. Secondly, as an ethical framework for the provision of health services on an equitable basis. Thirdly, as a fiscal framework for the construction of health care funding systems that enable cost-sharing and risk-pooling. Finally, as constituting the framework for the integration of a comprehensive range of upstream public health programmes within an overarching national health care system. Yet a commitment to achieving UHC continues to remain an aspirational one for many LIDCs, especially in Sub-Saharan Africa. This reflects the fragility of their national economies subject to the inevitable vagaries of the financial and market systems of global capitalism. Additionally, as the WHO has noted; '(T)he African region is also prone to natural disasters that have a human, economic and psychological impact. The types of energy and technologies are not modern or sustainable, especially in the rural areas, which generates challenges in ensuring the environment is healthy. On this basis countries in the WHO African Region need to make additional efforts and adopt new strategies and laws to improve their performance on the indicators for the health-related SDGs to be achieved by 2030' (WHO AFRO:2022;59).

The challenges faced by health systems in Sub-Saharan Africa

The rising incidence and prevalence of the 'double burden' of communicable and chronic disease is a considerable challenge for health systems in Sub-Saharan Africa. In 2017, the then Director-General of the WHO, Dr Tedros Adhanom Ghebreyesus, stated that, 'It is completely unacceptable that half the world still lacks coverage for the most essential health services; and it is unnecessary. A solution exists: universal health coverage (UHC) allowing everyone to obtain the health services they need, when and where they need them, without facing financial hardship' (WHO:2017). At one level this would appear to be an entirely uncontentious statement, yet it underplays the historic legacy of colonialism and associated economic 'underdevelopment' as experienced by many of these nations. This exploitative relationship continues to be manifested in high levels of international loan debt maintenance, the extraction and degradation of natural resources by multinational corporations, and the associated exacerbation of the already devastating impact of climate change on national infrastructures and food production.

According to a recent United Nations Development Programme report (UNDP:2023b), some 25 low-income countries now spend more than 20% of their national revenues on servicing national debt. This is the continuing legacy of the imposition of 'structural adjustment programmes' by the IMF and World Bank in the 1980s that included the requirement for deregulation and privatisation within national economies[2] in return for loans (Martin:2022). These on-going debt servicing costs have risen sharply since 2020 as the world's most powerful central banks have driven up interest rates in response to an inflation-led global economic crises. In human terms, the evident dysfunctionality of the global financial markets has led directly to an increase in the numbers of those now living below the $3.65-a-day UN poverty line. In the three years since 2020, an additional 165 million individuals globally have joined these ranks, constituting some 1.6 billion people or 20% of the world's population now living below this poverty line. According to the UNDP, 'On average, low-income countries are likely to allocate more than twice as much funding to servicing net interest payments as they do to social assistance, and 1.4 times more than to healthcare' (UNDP:2023b).

At this point it is useful to provide an overview of health expenditure trends, measured as a percentage of national GDP, in a sample of Sub-Saharan countries. Figure 6.1

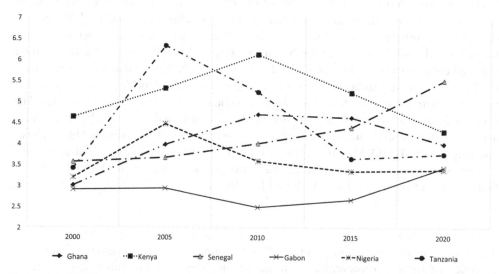

Figure 6.1 Health expenditure as % of GDP in selected African countries 2000–20 (Adapted from WHO Global database (2023a)).

shows some variation across the six countries (four in West Africa and two in East Africa) over two decade, but by 2020, just prior to the COVID-19 pandemic, health expenditure coalesces around the 4% of GDP mark. It is worth noting that the comparative figure for health expenditure in 2020 for HICs averaged around 12% of GDP. The 4% GDP figure in these six African countries represents a significant underfunding of services, manifested in the average of 2.9 doctors per 1,000 found in the WHO African Region, compared to 36.6 per 1,000 population in the WHO Europe Region (WHO AFRO:2022;140).

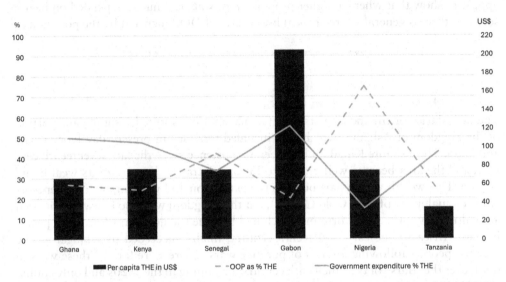

Figure 6.2 Measures of total health expenditure: selected African countries (Adapted from WHO Global database (2023a)).

This underfunding of health care across the WHO African Region in large part reflects the high average levels of national debt maintenance. This is evidenced in the proportion of state spending contributing to total health expenditure (THE) for six countries included in Figure 6.2. Gabon stands out because of its high per capita spending on health care at over US$ 200 compared to an average of US$ 70 in the other five countries. Gabon is a former French colony in West Africa, which until relatively recently has been a significant exporter of natural resources, including timber, manganese, and oil. Until 2017, before the global price fell, oil production accounted for up to 80% of the country's exports and 60% of state revenues. But by 2020, Gabon was running a fiscal deficit with a high level of inflation on goods and services (World Bank:2023a). With oil as a primary source of revenue, Gabon has historically been able to subsidise state health spending on health care up to a level of 50% of THE. This is reflected in the comparatively low level (20%) of individual out-of-pocket (OOP) payments, assessed as a percentage of THE. But the example of Gabon also demonstrates, that the extraction of oil and the other natural resources is inherently unsustainable and can result in long-term economic instability. This is the case not only in relation to the vagaries of oil prices in the global commodity markets, but the fact that it is a finite resource. Equally, the high levels of comparative per capita spending found in Gabon should not be interpreted as equating to a robust and equitable health system. The country is characterised by extreme levels of income inequality, demonstrating that the application of the per capita indicator for health spending alone can mask significant social differences in access to health care.

Like Gabon, Nigeria is also an important producer and exporter of oil, but these significant state revenues have not historically been reflected in the higher average levels of government health expenditure. OOP constitutes 75% of THE in Nigeria, and inevitably this regressive form of health spending disproportionately impacts on those living on or below the poverty line. While the data for Ghana, Kenya, Senegal, and Tanzania appear to show that where a higher proportion of state revenue is expended on health services, there is generally a reciprocal lower level of OOP incurred by the population.

****

Ghana: a brief historical and economic background

The boundaries of the modern state of Ghana once constituted a significant portion of the kingdom of Ashante, which also included territory in present-day Ivory Coast and Togo. The Ashante Kingdom had been in existence since the late seventeenth century, and the area became well known to European traders because of its wealth and culture. This wealth was in part built on the extraction and working of gold (hence its later colonial name of 'The Gold Coast'[3]), but the Kingdom was also known for its rich agriculture diversity. Great Britain, which had become the dominant European power in West Africa by the early nineteenth century, finally succeeded in subjugating the Ashante peoples following a series of punitive wars. There were four of these wars in total, over the course of the nineteenth century, beginning in the 1820s and only ending in 1895. As the 'Gold Coast', the territory of present-day Ghana was for over a century a British Imperial 'possession'.

Ghana became the first of Britain's former colonies in Africa to achieve majority rule independence. This followed a period of transition that saw a legislative assembly being established in 1952 as a constitutional halfway house. This assembly constituted a form of power-sharing with the resident British colonial governor on the path to eventual independence. Kwame Nkrumah,[4] who was the effective leader of the anti-colonial liberation movement in the Gold Coast, went on to become the head of this legislative assembly, and in March 1957, he became the democratically elected head of the first national government of the newly independent state of Ghana.

Today, Ghana has a population of some 30 million people, with an annual population growth rate of 2.13%, which is relatively low for Sub-Sahara Africa. Politically, it has a multi-party democratic system. Economically, there has been a slowdown in the rate of economic growth in recent years (a characteristic of many LIDCs), standing at 3.2% in 2022, which is expected to slow still further in the future. High inflation combined with this low growth rate has led to a rise in interest rates that has served to limit investment in the country, with the exception of its natural resource extractive industries. This state of affairs has further been compounded by the fact that the Ghanaian state's ability to generate demand in the economy has been 'weakened by lack of access to global capital markets and high debt service obligations' (World Bank:2023b).

In their contribution to a collection of papers published to coincide with the Sixtieth Anniversary of Ghanaian independence, de-Graft Aikins and Koram (2017) have highlighted the ways in which the health status and quality of life of Ghanaians has developed since independence. They begin by noting the fact that at the time of independence, the major challenges faced by the health system were infectious diseases, high rates of maternal mortality, and a range of child health conditions arising from poverty and lack of widespread immunisation programmes. Sixty years on, Ghana, like many other LICD countries, now faces the 'double burden' of infectious and chronic non-communicable diseases (NCDs). This outcome, according to the authors, reflects the demographic and socio-economic changes that have occurred over this period: '(L)ife expectancy has increased. Fertility rates have declined. While the country remains predominantly youthful, the population of older adults aged 60 and above has grown. The country has become more urbanized with reported improvements in socio-economic and nutrition status. Yet there is a growing population of poor disenfranchised urban slum communities. Across communities and households, there is a co-existence of over-nutrition and under-nutrition attributed to food market globalization and changing agricultural policies and practices' (de-Graft Aikins & Koram:2017;365). While there has been a decline in childhood mortality and maternal mortality rates since the Millennium, women from poorer families and particularly those living in more rural regions of the country are still much more likely to experience complications in pregnancy. Neglected tropical diseases (NTDs) continue to be prevalent and disproportionately impact on the elderly.

The double burden of disease found in Ghana and many other Sub-Saharan countries reflects the fact that these countries do not easily conform to the 'standard', or more accurately, the Western conceptualisation of the 'epidemiological transition'.[5] The transition from predominantly acute to chronic patterns of disease has been much more protracted in LICs, which has had serious implications for the structure and functioning of their health systems. Health systems such as Ghana's, 'have typically been developed to address infectious diseases of short duration and have struggled to provide equitable healthcare to their most vulnerable citizens' (de-Graft Aikins & Koram:2017;369). It should also be noted that while mental health disorders are just as prevalent in LIDCs as in HICs, but in the case of Ghana and many other African health systems, there has been a general neglect of the treatment and management of these disorders within the population.[6]

Institutional processes and the development of the Ghanaian health system

Post-independence Ghana inherited a mish-mash of a health care infrastructure from the British. This consisted of a collection of Christian mission hospitals and health centres that were located primarily within the capital, Accra, as well as along the southern coastal region, but with only a limited infrastructure within the country's hinterland. The legacy of colonial underdevelopment could only be addressed through a process of state investment given that reliance on private market forces was not an option at the time of independence. Yet as Crawford Young has noted, this period of the late 1950s, when independence from colonial rule was becoming a reality, also 'coincided with the zenith of confidence in state-led development' (Young:2004;29). This was the period when national welfare states were being consolidated in Western countries, five-year strategic plans were being implemented by the centralised states of the Communist bloc in Eastern Europe as well as in China. Young cites the Ghanaian

President, Kwame Nkrumah writing in 1962, that 'most of our development so far has had to be carried out by the government itself. There is no other way out' (Young:2004;30).

Health policy in newly independent Ghana was driven by a post-colonial political idealism, and one of the key goals of the government was to expand and improve the health care infrastructure through state-directed planning and funding. The primary policy goal was to institute a system of free health care in order to achieve an equitable and affordable provision of health care. Some 35 new health centres were constructed, dispersed across the country, while the first medical school in the country was established in 1964. Capacity for the training of nurses and other groups of health care professionals also expanded at this time, but the initial capital investment in training, health facilities and medical equipment could not be sustained over a longer period by state tax revenues alone. This situation reflected the essential fragility of the inherited colonial economy, manifest in inconsistent and limited revenue streams. Ultimately, it was this economic instability combined with later fiscal mismanagement and endemic corruption amongst state officials that led onto the military coup of 1966, which overthrew the democratically elected Nkrumah government.

Over the next course of the next quarter of a century, Ghana witnessed a merry-go-round of democratically elected governments being reinstated then being toppled in turn by a military coup (five in total). At the same time, Ghana increasingly became submerged in a national debt crises that lasted up until the early 1990s. The country was subjected to the imposition of the so-called 'Structural Adjustment Programs' imposed by the World Bank and IMF in exchange for debt-relief. Military-led governments proved to be no less able than civilian ones in navigating these global financial restrictions. Ultimately, both civilian and military governments adopted the austerity policies required of them by the IMF, this had the consequence of seriously eroding the effectiveness of the health care services and widening social and health inequalities (de-Graft Aikins & Koram:2017;371). Some attempts were made by government to maintain levels of investment in health care services through raising fees, prescription charges, and other OOPs, but this inevitably led onto a widening of social inequity in health provision as services became prohibitively expensive for the majority of the population.

It was not until the establishment of a new constitution in 1992 that the long sequence of military rule interspersed with short-lived elected governments finally came to an end. This was also the period when improvement began to occur in rates of economic growth and development, in large part because the IMF belatedly recognised the 'miscalculations' it had made in its imposition of austerity budgets in return for debt relief back in the 1980s. By 1999, the IMF was formally acknowledging, 'the importance of protecting or increasing social expenditures during adjustment ... (with) targets for health and education spending now routinely part of ESAF-supported programs' (IMF:1999). The early 1990s also saw an expansion of health service provision in both secondary care hospital-based provision and primary care services. This reflected a significant increase in capital investment by non-state (charitable 'missions' and voluntary providers) and private health care sectors. Yet this expansion of private and charitable health service provision simply reinforced the imbalanced structure of health care provision in the country. The more cost-efficient and equitable policy option of public investment in upstream disease prevention programmes was eschewed. In part this was because the private health sector had little or no monetary incentive to engage in community-based public health programmes, this being an area of health provision where significant profits could not easily be made. The paradox here was that Ghana was one of the early signatories to the 1978 WHO Ata Declaration on public health widely known as the 'Health for All' strategy. Clause V of the declaration stated that: 'Governments have a responsibility for the health of their people which can be fulfilled only by the provision of adequate health and social measures .... (P)rimary health care is the key to attaining this target as part of development in the spirit of social justice' (WHO:1978;3). Despite its formal commitment to these principles, few public health initiatives were ever initiated in Ghana, from the first military coup in 1966 until the return to democratic governance in the 1990s.

Since the late 1990s, the Ghana Health service has looked to develop innovative methods for delivering primary care, largely due to the constraints of its limited budget expenditure. This approach is formally known as Community Health Planning Services (CHPS). This programme has sought to utilise trained community health workers to provide some basic clinical as well as preventative health services, including the delivery of the immunisation programme in the under-served districts and regions within the country. The programme has had some success over the last two decades and has since expanded into urban areas. Nevertheless, the objective of providing extensive equitable primary care has been undermined by financial, resource and logistical challenges (de-Graft Aikins & Koram:2017;374). This situation draws attention to Geoffrey Rose's authoritive notion of the 'prevention paradox', that 'a measure that brings large benefits to the community offers little to each participating individual' (1981;1847). That is, for community primary and prevention health programmes to be effective they should involve the participation of as large as proportion of the population as possible. For Rose, targeted disease prevention programmes that only focus medical intervention on those identified as at 'high risk' is not an effective strategy, as the 'not-yet-at-high-risk' population groups miss out on the benefits of early intervention.

Ghanaian state spending on health, equated to less than 1% of total GDP, in the decades prior to the new Millennium. Since then, there has been an upward trajectory but with some downturns reflecting trends in the global financial markets, so that by 2020 state spending constituted some 2% of GDP (WHO AFRO:2023a). Yet the increasing reliance on private market investment remains problematic for the long-term sustainability of the Ghanaian national health care system. Some 40% of health care facilities are privately owned, including hospitals, clinics, pharmacies, and diagnostic laboratory facilities. According to the Ghana Living Standards Survey (GLSS7) carried out in 2017, over 50% of health care consultations are accessed through the private health sector (GSS:2017). This state of affairs was particularly problematic during the COVID-19 epidemic when a comprehensive national public health response was most required (Nimako et al:2020).

If an over-reliance on PHI and OOP payments (colloquially known in Ghana as the 'cash and carry' system) is problematic for the achievement of health equity, then what has changed in relation to alternative sources of pooled health care funding in the intervening years? In 2003, the New Patriotic Party, which had come into power three years earlier, fulfilled its electoral promise to establish a National Health Insurance Scheme (NHIS). The stated objective of the scheme was to 'provide financial risk protection against healthcare services for all persons resident in Ghana' (NHIA:2023).

Although in principle all citizens are potentially eligible for insurance cover, NHIS is neither a universal nor compulsory state health insurance scheme. It is financed primarily through the National Health Insurance Levy, a 2.5% value-added tax (VAT) on all goods and services, combined with a social insurance (SSNIT) deduction from salaried occupations also at a rate of 2.5%, as well as direct premiums paid by those in 'informal' or non-salaried work. Ghana is the only country in Africa to finance its health insurance scheme primarily through VAT. The advantage of relying on VAT as a supplement to the employee levy is that the price of goods and services automatically keeps pace with economic growth (where wages may not), and so NHIS has been able to sustain its share of total government spending. Utilising VAT revenue to finance health care 'constitutes an implicit subsidy for basic care, and it provides a basis for pooling risks and costs at the national level, which prevents the scheme fragmentation experienced by many other countries' (Wang et al:2017;17).

As of 2020, there were approximately 12 million active members of the NHIS representing over 50% of the population, this number represents an incremental increase in enrolments into the scheme since its inception. The NHIS covers 95% of diagnosed conditions and has no cost-sharing requirements. It covers all outpatient, inpatient, and emergency care costs, and the list of excluded conditions is explicitly defined. NHIS members also pay no OOP costs for services or pharmaceuticals (NHIA:2023). Here it should be noted that those who are not enrolled in the scheme, nearly half the population, have to pay the full cost of any medical treatment OOP. The tariffs or payments received by health care providers for treating NHIS recognised diagnosis-related groups differ by forms of ownership and facility type. Private sector providers receive the highest tariffs and capitation rates to compensate for their lack of public funding, while public service providers (including the Christian Missions) receive funding directly from the Ghanaian Ministry of Health. Additionally, while the VAT revenue source of funding has its advantages, it has one major disadvantage, which is that revenue does not increase as coverage expands. In recent years, the growth of claims expenditures has outpaced the growth of NHIS revenue causing a sizable deficit for the scheme. Several factors have contributed to this increase in claims, a widening of the population now covered by the scheme, an increase in health service utilisation (including the children of NIHS members), and rising private provider costs (Wang et al:2017;27).

An interesting aspect of the Ghanaian NHIS is why half the population (48% as of 2020) are not enrolled in the scheme, given that the individual costs of membership are not relatively high compared to national health insurance schemes that exist elsewhere across the globe. A recent study carried out by Owusu Sarkodie (2021) looked into this question, utilising data from the Ghana Living Standards Survey (GLSS 7). It was found that many of those who were not enrolled in the scheme worked in the informal sector of the economy, and so live with irregular sources of income. As such, many were put off enrolling because of the requirement to make regular premium payments. A lack of trust in the NHIS was also cited as a reason for not enrolling, many preferring to chance the risk of ill-health, and if this does occur, to then rely on OOPs for the treatment they required. Others preferred to utilise traditional healers (discussed below), a much more affordable source of treatment.

A relatively recent systematic review of both qualitative and quantitative research has examined the impact of the implementation of the NHIS for health care in Ghana.

The review concluded that the Ghanaian NHIS, almost uniquely amongst Sub-Saharan countries, has the potential to providing access to health care for all sections of the Ghanaian population. Yet after nearly 20 years of existence, the scheme has not succeeded in protecting the whole population from the 'negative consequences of OOP health care costs' and that 'national coverage or UHC is far from reach at this pace'. The scheme now faces the significant challenge of addressing, 'poor coverage; poor quality of care; corruption and ineffective governance; poor stakeholder participation; lack of clarity on concepts in the policy; intense political influence; and poor financing' (Christmals & Aidam:2020;1899).

Decentralising the Ghanaian health care system?

In the first three decades following independence, Ghana was characteristically a top-down centralised system of state control, often under military command. Since the instigation of the Fourth Republic constitution in 1992, there has been a gradual recognition of the need for greater decentralisation of state authority in a country marked by significant regional differences. This situation is not unique to Ghana, and a process of decentralisation is apparent in several other post-colonial countries in Africa, including Kenya (discussed below). The logic of decentralising administrative responsibility for health care services, alongside the promotion of the CHPS initiative described above, is that in principle it enables a greater degree of local managerial autonomy which may be more responsive to local needs and meet equity goals. However, the outcomes of the process of decentralising health care provision in Ghana have been somewhat mixed.

One study conducted in the Upper West Region of Ghana found that in practice the commitment to devolving autonomy to local managers was limited, serving only to reinforce the status quo of the national state in ultimately determining health resource allocations. It was also found that decentralisation, locally known as the 'deconcentrated system', provided 'little or no mechanism for local governance popular participation in health sector decision-making ... (and) the role of local managers is limited to making recommendations to national level for whatever action is required' (Sumah:2014;49). Even as overall investment in the health care system has increased, the uneven regional distribution of health resources (and this includes health care professionals) that was a defining, characteristic of provision during the colonial era, continues. Here the centrifugal pull of the capital Accra is a major factor, abetted by the existence of a 'culture of parallel health care provision', wherein clinical specialists offer private consultation services alongside their formally paid state services (de-Graft Aikins & Koram:2017;374). The Nkrumah government banned this practice in the 1960s, but following the military coup the practice returned. Today this parallel system continues to exist, its impact exacerbated by the expansion of the private health sector, with significant implications for the achievement of equitable access to high-quality health care as well as the overall cost-effectiveness of the health system. This is a country where in 2023, some 24% of the national population were identified as living in poverty (and over 35% in rural areas), assessed on the basis of the Oxford Poverty and Human Development Initiative 'Multidimensional Poverty Index' (OPHI:2023).

The migration of health care professionals:
'Push-Pull' factors in Ghana

A key challenge for health systems across the African continent has been to retain their health care professional staff in response to what has euphemistically referred to as the 'brain drain'. More accurately stated, this is the process understood as a 'push-pull' migratory effect that operates at a global level. The 'pull' factors correspond to the ever increasing demands on high-income health systems of 'ageing populations' that has followed the demographic shift towards larger numbers of older people living longer and with chronic conditions.[7] As LIDCs started to build their own medical educational capacity to train local health care professionals, so health systems in wealthier countries began to recruit these staff to fill their own vacancies. Health systems in HICs have the capacity to pay higher wages, provide improved conditions of employment, and offer professional career development pathways. A further 'pull' factor for former British colonies such as Ghana and Kenya is the use of a common language as well as similarities in professional training systems, which had made working in the UK an especially attractive proposition (Dovlo:2003;4). The 'push' factors in countries such as Ghana include the relatively low level of salaries for professional roles; low levels of work satisfaction that reflects the limited availability of the modern equipment to enable these professionals to perform at the level they are trained for; and the perception of a health system characterised by poor governance manifest as a lack of hierarchical accountability. On top of these factors are relatively high levels of political instability which in turn have contributed to the decision of health professionals to migrate.

Ghana saw a steady decline in the ratio of health professionals to population from the 1970s onwards. But it was only from the late 1990s that the government recognised the need to take action, and began to direct additional resources towards expanding the number of training places for nurses, doctors, and other health professionals allied to medicine, plus an overall increase in salaries. But the push-pull factors driving the economic migration of health care professions have not abated. As recently as June 2023, the BBC News ran a story that cited a figure of 1200 Ghanaian nurses joining the UK Nursing Registry over the course of the previous year. The BBC article went onto state that: '(A)lthough the UK says active recruitment in Ghana is not allowed, social media means nurses can easily see the vacancies available in NHS trusts. They can then apply for those jobs directly. Ghana's dire economic situation acts as a big push factor'. The Deputy Head of Nursing Services at Cape Coast Municipal Hospital, Caroline Agbodza, is quoted in this BBC News report as saying that she had seen 22 nurses leave for the UK in the last year: "*All our critical care nurses, our experienced nurses, have gone. So we end up having nothing – no experienced staff to work with. Even if the government recruits, we have to go through the pain of training nurses again*". Smaller clinics are particularly affected by staff migration because even one nurse leaving a small health centre can have a large knock-on effect ... At Kwaso healthcare centre near the city of Kumasi, Mercy Asare Afriyie explained that she was hoping to find a job in the UK soon, "*The exodus of nurses is not going to stop because of our poor conditions of service. Our salary is nothing to write home about and in two weeks you spend it. It's from hand to mouth*". Ghanaian nurses told the BBC that in the UK they could earn more than seven times what they are receiving in Ghana' (BBC:2023).

Yet from a UK perspective (hence the BBC News interest), what is perhaps most significant about this recent update on the economic migration of health professionals from Ghana is the impact of Brexit. The migration policies of the UK have become more severe for asylum seekers in recent years, but pragmatically more flexible in relation to qualified professional staff, since the withdrawal from the European Union (EU) on January 31, 2020. It was on this note that the BBC News story concluded, quoting the WHO's Director of Health Workforce, Jim Campbell as follows: 'The labour market is extremely competitive around the world and, having closed off the potential labour market from European freedom of movement, what we're seeing is the consequences of that in terms of attracting people from the Commonwealth and other jurisdictions' (BBC:2023).

****

Kenya: a brief historical and economic background

Kenya is also a former British Imperial African 'possession' located in East Africa. The country gained its independence in 1963, but only following a long drawn-out struggle marked by violence and political suppression.

The British Colonial Office established what it called the 'East Africa Protectorate' in 1895, a territory that stretched from the Indian Ocean through to the Great Lakes, largely to exploit the potential of the rich agricultural lands that had long sustained subsistence farming for many communities. The initial focus for Imperial exploitation was the coastal regions because of the ease of access for shipping, via the historic port of Mombasa. But with the development of a railway network in 1901, the hinterland became more accessible, enabling the commercial development of cash crops such as tea and coffee grown solely for the export market. Over time, the indigenous peoples of this region saw their traditional forms of clan and tribal-based governance of land management replaced by a system of District and Provincial Commissioners. This imposed authority was composed of British Civil Servants, with a Crown-appointed Governor at its apex; with indigenous East Africans effectively excluded from any possibility of political self-determination. Alongside the denial of legal and social rights, the British colonial state engaged in, 'a cultural conquest which destroyed or attempted to destroy the African ways of living and belief systems, religions, social assimilation patterns and customs' (Mburu:1981;521).

Kenya, as was the case in nearly all the African territories controlled by European colonisers in the late nineteenth and early twentieth centuries, was effectively forced to pay for its own subjugation (Young:2004;26). In the region now controlled by the British Empire, surplus value generated from the production and trade in commodities was historically low, this reflected the preexisting agricultural system of production which primarily operated as a subsistence economy: '(I)n the absence of any significant pre-existing revenue flows (that could be appropriated), the solution was to monetize the African subject by the imposition of head taxes and fiscal extraction in kind through forced labour' (Young:2004;26). This 'low-cost' colonial model characterised British rule until after the Second World War, marked by a minimalist social infrastructure that stood in contrast to the primacy accorded to the exploitation and export of natural resources. Following the Second World War, and up to and including Independence in

1963, there was an exponential increase in commodity production in Kenya, which is sometimes termed 'the second colonial occupation'. This late period of colonial exploitation resulted in a legacy of 'widespread environmental degradation. Forest concessions, which were granted to individuals and companies led to massive deforestation. Colonial enterprises destroyed local industries' (Ndege:2009;3).

Civil society in colonial-era Kenya was also distinguished by the institutionalisation of an ideology of European racial superiority. At the end of the nineteenth century, the Colonial Office instigated a policy of encouraging and facilitating the migration of large numbers of people from pre-partition Imperial India to East Africa. These new migrants were predominately indentured labourers brought in specifically to construct the railway network, but they also included amongst their number some business traders, as well as clerks to oil the machinery of the colonial bureaucracy. Since the sixteenth century, Indian merchants and sailors had played a significant role in the Indian Ocean trading networks that stretched from the East African coast, through Arabia all the way to the Indian sub-continent itself. But this imposed migration process was of a different order. During the colonial era, the Indian community or East African Asians as they were later to be categorised, served an important social function as an 'ethnic minority buffer' between the British rulers and the indigenous Africans. The living standards and the rights of East African Asians reflected this 'divide-and-rule' colonial strategy of control. The 'in-betweener' status for people of an Asian heritage had the long-term consequence of making them targets for both ethnic and class divide resentment, and this remained the case in the post-colonial era until relatively recently.[8]

The political struggle for independence from British rule was led by the Kenya African National Union (KANU), a nationalist political party founded in 1944, following the legalisation of Kenyan political organisations. The legalisation of African political parties was the direct result of the colonial government's concern to avoid confrontation over the demand for national self-determination. It was not a coincidence that this legalisation occurred at a time when Kenya's economy, as well as its geopolitical position, was crucial to the British war effort. By the early 1950s, alongside the political campaign for independence, the colonial settler communities in the rural hinterland were confronted by an uprising of peasant farmers seeking the return of tribal homelands and the establishment of equitable land rights for Africans. This struggle mutated into a bitter guerrilla war led by the Land and Freedom Army (known disparagingly as the 'Mau Mau'), which was eventually violently and cruelly suppressed by British Army forces in 1952. By 1960, Britain had effectively conceded that Kenya would become an independent self-governing country and embarked on a programme of land reform while it was still the colonial power. Anticipating post-independence nationalisation of settler-owned plantations, the British colonial authorities established a land transfer scheme that has since been described as, 'one of the most generous compensations for political losses of landownership known in economic history. But it was to be independent Kenya and not Britain, which was to end up shouldering the bulk of the costs' (Leo:1981;216).

The post-independence history of Kenya is described in the following section in the context of the challenges associated with the development of its health care system. But to provide a concise summery, Kenya today has a multi-party democratic system, and no one political party or coalition of parties has held office for more than one term of office since the ending of the effective single party rule of KANU from the time of independence in 1963 up until 2002. Over the past two decades the Kenyan political system has been dominated by party coalitions that 'remain fundamentally ethnic and regional machines...scrambled together on the eve of elections to win power ... never having stabilized into coherent political parties with national reach and resonance' (Khadiagala:2023).

Today, Kenya has a population of some 54 million people with an annual population growth of 1.9%, which is relatively low for Sub-Sahara Africa. Life expectancy at birth is 61 years. 76% of the population has access to electricity, and 31% have access to safely managed sanitation (World Bank:2022). The economic growth rate averaged nearly 5% per year from 2015 up until the COVID-19 pandemic in 2020, and it was largely due to the resilience of the agricultural export sector that any contraction in the economy during this period was minimal. The economic growth rate has since returned to 5% per annum as of 2022, with GDP per capita average incomes at $2,100 (World Bank:2022). The latest World Bank economic outlook recognises that Kenya continues to experience key development challenges that include: '(P)overty, youth unemployment, transparency and accountability, climate change, continued weak private sector investment, and the vulnerability of the economy to internal and external shocks' (World Bank:2023c). In mid-2024, Kenya experienced nationwide protests over government tax rises, political corruption, and widening social and ethnic inequalites.

Institutional processes and the development of the Kenyan health system

As was also the case in colonial Ghana, the influence of the Christian Missions, which first established themselves within Kenya at the end of the nineteenth century had a distorting effect on the development of health service provision within the country. The history of the relationship between Christian missionaries of all denominations and the expansion of European colonies in Africa was a complimentary one, so that in the colonies, 'healing went hand-in-hand with proselytization' (Mburu:1981;523). By the 1920s, missionary medical services were the primary source of health care for Africans and Asians in Kenya, although these services were neither systematically distributed across the country nor of a high quality. Some health services were organised by the colonial authority themselves, but these were exclusively for the White settlers. Nevertheless, from the early years of colonisation it was understood that the endemic communicable diseases of the region also carried a threat to the European settlers.[9] Effective control of diseases such as malaria, cholera, and blackwater fever (a complication of malaria) would always be ineffective unless the colonisers also invested in the health of their African employees; '(I)n short, the medical system, vigorously instituted was designed to benefit the European immigrants. The Africans were just a necessary problem of that maintenance process' (Mburu:1981;522).

By the time of the Second World War, the colonial state operating a three-tier system of health care, each serving a particular ethnic group. There were European hospitals, which also contained lower standard 'Asiatic Wards', and there were hospital exclusively for Africans run largely by the missions: 'Public medical services were largely confined to the urban coastal centres, and those hinterland areas that were deemed to have acquiesced to colonial rule' (Mburu:1981;524). This racialised hierarchical organisation of health services was to be maintained in the years following independence, with the key difference being that the colonial-era racial divide in provision effectively became a socio-economic class divide. The inequity of provision as between rural and urban areas has also continued.[10]

Following independence, the new Kenyan government enthusiastically committed itself to a pathway of economic and social development focused on the elimination of poverty, disease, and illiteracy. A cornerstone of this programme was the goal of establishing a universal 'free health for all' policy. This would necessitate a significant expansion of the existing health care infrastructure and levels of provision, closely linked to the construction of a sustainable health funding system. This commitment was gradually undermined and eroded by political and social turmoil, a dramatic increase in the population, and the systemic weaknesses of Kenya's economy as a major legacy of colonialism. The decades that followed independence saw an increasing reliance by the government on borrowing, drawing down loans from the international financial markets. But these loans came with attendant terms and conditions that mandated market-orientated structural reforms within the economy, seeking to limit an interventionary role for the state, as well as strict debt repayment schedules with onerous penalties for defaulting.

Health care services in post-independence Kenya have been funded through a mixed economy of health care financing. At independence, Kenya inherited a colonial system where user fees for health care were the norm, this effectively limited access and utilisation of services for the majority of the population. Consistent with its declared programme to eradicate poverty, the nationalist-led KANU government formally abolished user fees and established the National Insurance Health Fund (NIHF) in 1966 as a separate department within the Ministry of Health; this is now the oldest national state insurance scheme in Africa. The declared objective in establishing this pooled insurance fund was to reduce levels of health inequity and widen access to health care provision. The NIHF was developed as a compulsory scheme for all salaried employees in formal sector of the economy whose income exceeded a minimum level. The scheme was designed to be self-funding, with no facility for state budgetary support. Yet the majority of those of working age were employed within the informal sector of the economy, and while they were in principle able to voluntarily opt into the insurance scheme, in practice they effectively found it was out of their reach both financially as well as in practical terms given the scheme required regular monthly contributions.

Two decades later, as the price to pay for an increasing dependency on international monetary loans to offset an under-performing economy and rising unemployment, the Kenyan government made the decision to reintroduce user fees in order to reduce state expenditure on health care. At the same time, it reversed its previous commitment to the achievement of UHC by encouraging the expansion of private health care provision. The imposition of austerity budgets and the privatisation of state assets was the price extracted by the IMF and global commercial banks for these loans. It was not until 2004 that user fees for accessing the very basic health services provided in dispensaries and health centres were removed (yet again). Then in 2007, user fees were abolished in all public sector health facilities, resulting in a gradual increase in service utilisation rates. The caveat being that public sector health care facilities were not widespread, so that many in the population continued to rely on the private health sector and OOPs. So it was that by 2011, the level of risk-pooling[11] via the NIHF scheme continued to be minimal with just 10% of the population covered. While at the same time, the health care needs of 600,000 of the wealthiest citizens of Kenya were funded through private health insurance premiums. The wealthy families generally lived within the capital Nairobi and had easy access to local private health facilities (Chuma & Okunga:2011;6).

In 2014, the Kenyan government was finally forced to respond to the increasing political pressure to fundamentally reform the system of health care funding. It produced a road map for the achievement of UHC, entitled the 'Kenya Health Policy 2014–30' (Kenya MoH:2014). A key pillar of this strategy was a series of reforms that sought to expand the population coverage of the NIHF. Contribution rates were increased for members in both the informal and formal employment sectors, with the quid pro quo being an expansion of benefit entitlements to include outpatient care plus a range of medical care 'specialised packages'. For health care providers (both private and public sector), there was also an upward revision of payments for care services. Yet, a review of the impact of these reforms conducted three years after their implementation was largely negative and concluded that rather than improving the quality of care and widening equity in provision, they had only served to further 'compromise' accessibility of the health system (Barasa et al:2018). This review further found that health insurance rates had increased by as much as 100% for many in the formal sector, and over 200% for many of those in the informal sector. The outcome of these increases was that the NIHF scheme became even more unaffordable for many. In addition, the quid pro quo aspects of the 2014 reforms that involved expansion of available services for those in the scheme could not be delivered in practice because of shortages of equipment and trained staff. Yet the private sector was able to expand its range of services to some former NIHF members, although largely restricted to those resident in urban areas (Barasa et al:2018). Nevertheless, by 2018, the NIHF had at least managed to achieve near universal coverage amongst those in salaried employment in the formal sector of the economy, but opting-in amongst those in the informal sector continued to remain low. Overall, the reforms achieved an increase in insurance coverage equivalent to just 19% of the total population of the country.

Decentralising the Kenyan health care system?

This section focuses on the attempts by the Kenyan government to more equitable manage the infrastructure and levels of service provision across the country, beyond the reforms to the system of funding described above. A major development in this process has been the shift to a decentralised model of health governance.

In 2010, following a period of political and social turmoil, the government embarked on a redrafting of the national Constitution, the supreme law of the country. This was seen as necessary in order to reduce the power of the executive branch of government, a legacy of the post-colonial constitution and the one-party rule that had characterised the political system in Kenya until 2002. This post-independence command-and-control centralised state structure was widely held responsible for the failure to recognise the popular discontent resulting from the widening gap in social and ethnic inequalities that led to a national outbreak of violent conflict following the National Elections in 2007. The formal objective in reducing the power of the executive was to devolve central authority and to guarantee the rights of women and minorities. A national referendum on the proposed changes resulted in a 68% majority in favour of constitutional reform that was signed into law in 2010. The new Constitution formally separated the judicial, legislative, and executive branches of the state, and replaced the federal structure of government with a two-tier devolved system of government. The first tier was to be the national government, and the second tier was the new state authorities representing the 52 counties of the country. To facilitate the 'levelling-up' of the more economically deprived rural counties, an 'equalization fund' was also established, equivalent to 0.5% of national revenue.

Included in the programme of regional devolution, and directly linked to the government's long-term strategic commitment to achieving UHC, was the decision in 2012 to re-organise the national structure of health care management and planning. The budgetary allocation for health care was now devolved to the 52 counties, with the national government tasking these regional authorities with ensuring the successful implementation of the 2014–30 national health strategy. The Kenyan Ministry of Health has claimed that in the decade following this re-organisation, the national budget for the health sector increased by 200% as a percentage of total government spending (Kenya MoH:2022;vii). Yet national state health spending measured as a percentage of THE has *not* increased in line with this commitment and has remained stagnant at below 50% THE over this period. Little progress has been made in cost-sharing and state subsidising of health care, a key determining factor in the failure to make progress on UHC. Devolving control to regional councils has led to, 'the absence of a centralized, systematic and inclusive process through which this (UHC) agenda can be driven … (and subsequently) a lack of definition of the values and trade-offs competing for health resources within Kenya's limited fiscal space, making it difficult to implement meaningful resource and strategic investment into health policy goals' (Oraro-Lawrence & Wyss:2020;8). As of 2022, OOPs continue to constitute a significant proportion (26%) of Kenyan THE (WHO:2022).

A decade on, a review of the impact of the 2010 constitutional changes concluded that the shift to devolved government continued to face significant challenges. These included: '(I)ncoherent national policymaking and leadership, weak technical capacity at county level, poorly implemented or non-existent mechanisms for public consultation, and a lack of gender-disaggregated data on which to base policymaking. Despite these obstacles, some counties have made real progress. But overall the impact of devolution on equality has been limited …. (T)here is a glaring gap between policy commitments and actual investments by county governments' (Kimani:2020;1).

****

The role of traditional medicine in the Ghanaian and Kenyan health system

Traditional forms of medicine are best understood as focused on achieving a balance between the individual, their local community and the surrounding environment: 'With a few exceptions, the traditional doctor shares the belief system of the patient. Indeed, the doctor and the patient belong to the same *integrated* socio-cultural group supported by an established framework of social norms' (Mburu:1981;522 – *italics in original*). The traditional forms of medicine that are to be found in Africa and elsewhere across the globe have until relatively recently, sat uncomfortably alongside 'modern' biomedical systems. The 'modern' health care systems that developed in Europe and North America towards the end of the nineteenth century largely eschewed any recognition of the implicit worth of traditional forms of medicine, citing a lack of any evidence-base for many of its practises. Indeed, the early history of European colonialism is marked by the attempt to suppress traditional medical practices in favour of 'modernity', although that principle rarely extended to the point of actually providing 'modern' health care facilities for indigenous populations. Yet today, health policy decision-makers, particularly in low- and medium-income countries, are more open to the contribution that traditional medicine can make to health care provision and population health outcomes.

Ghana and Kenya are examples of the attempt to build an effective strategy of integrating traditional medicine within a national health system. These two countries are not isolated instances of this approach, they both signed-up to, and in Ghana's case preceded, the early promotion of this strategy by the WHO that emerged as was one of the many outcomes of the 1978 Alma-Ata 'Health for All' conference and declaration (also discussed above with reference to Ghana's health prevention strategy). The rationale that underpinned the promotion of integration was that traditional and complimentary medicine (T&CM) as it became termed, was a more affordable, accessible, and acceptable option for many local communities. As such it was seen as having a great potential to contribute to disease prevention strategies. Many health systems around the globe, and with the support of the WHO, now began to consider how to take up this challenge.

Two decades after the Alma-Ata Declaration, the WHO reiterated its T&CM principles in its strategy document, *Traditional Practitioners as Primary Health Care Workers* (WHO:1995). Here it was stated that: '(T)he Western system of healing has not replaced but has augmented indigenous health systems. This is because traditional healing is deeply embedded in wider belief systems and remains integral part of the lives of most people' (WHO:1995;2). The strategy provided examples of health systems, including that of Ghana, which had attempted to integrate traditional medicine and to assess the issues that were then emerging. A further two decades down the line, the WHO published an update and reassessment of its integration strategy (WHO:2013). The purpose of this publication was to set out explicit guidelines and recommendations for 'the appropriate integration, regulation and supervision traditional practitioners, and will be useful to countries wishing to develop a proactive policy towards this important, and often vibrant and expanding part of health care' (WHO:2013;7). Even more recently in 2022, the WHO has produced a series of standards and terminological guidance for a wide range of traditional forms of medicine practiced across the globe, although not necessarily integrated with biomedical health care systems.

Ghana was one of the early adopters of the movement to integrate traditional medicine into its biomedical health care system, as a 'complimentary' medical practice. In 1961, just four years after achieving Independence, the Nkrumah government was influential in the establishment of the Ghana Psychic and Traditional Healers Association. In the 1970s, a centre for the study of safe and efficacious herbal medicines was also developed, and this served to provide bioscientific legitimacy to the practise of traditional medicine. The Traditional and Alternative Medicine Directorate was established by the Ministry of Health in 1991 and given the responsibility of coordinating the formal integration of T&CM within the Ghanaian health system. Subsequently however, the government has been criticised for providing only lip service to their policy because it has failed to provide the support and resources required to make integration a practical proposition. Few of the regulations necessary to ensure compliance with best T&CM practice have ever been implemented. The lack of regulatory structures is also seen as having a negative impact on health outcomes. This is because traditional medicine, 'is a major driver of "healer shopping" and therefore of late presentation to biomedical facilities, and so is often implicated in avoidable disease complications and deaths' (de-Graft Aikins & Koram:2017;372).

A rather more positive assessment of the contribution of TC&M can be found in a relatively recent study of the relationships of trust that exist between traditional healers and biomedical professionals in the rural Northern Region of Ghana (Krah et al:2018). In this qualitative study, several challenges to the successful integration of traditional healers and biomedical staff were identified. These included a limited understanding about the degree to which a framework of traditional healing was integrated within local cultures. This lack of understanding was found to be strongly linked to the discriminatory attitudes that were held by many health professionals towards healers, who were often regarded as being 'backward'. It was also found that the high turnover of medical staff in this rural region served to undermine the establishment of long-term relationships of trust with traditional healers. However, the study did go on to identify opportunities for integration. These included the recognition that healers are trusted within the rural communities and so are able to maintain an infrastructure of care that can play an important role in cross-referring patients to medical facilities. The study also identified a willingness of at least some medical professional staff to collaborate with certain healer groups, although not all, because of their recognised skills for example in bone-healing or herbalism. It was also found that many traditional healers expressed their eagerness to develop their own biomedical knowledge in order to collaborate more closely with biomedical clinical staff. It was on the basis of their findings that the authors of the study concluded that 'power-sensitive relationships' should be encouraged and constructed between traditional healers and biomedical staff in the field. This would be a much more positive alternative to viewing the role of healers within the health system as restricted to referring people onto biomedical facilities. Insufficient 'attention is paid to actual dialogue with healers …. (who) should be appreciated and recognised symbolically and materially … accompanied by a communication strategy aimed at explaining and promoting integration and educating stakeholders' (Krah et al:2018;162).

It was not until the early 1980s that the Kenyan Ministry of Health fully committed itself to the integration of T&CM within the health care system. This decision was strongly influenced by the requirement to expand health coverage into rural areas where there was an acute unfulfilled health need. Traditional midwives were recruited to work in state health care facilities for this purpose having undergone a process of prior training in order to 'professionalise' their traditional knowledge and practice (Mwabu:1995;249). Nevertheless, it has been argued that the health system has simply co-opted traditional healers because they are relatively affordable and accessible in rural areas, in order to mask the fact that the majority of Kenyans are effectively disenfranchised from access to high-quality health care facilities because of the high levels of poverty and job security (Wamai:2009). In 2003, partly as a consequence of the failure to effectively regulate T&CM healers, a new legislative framework, the Traditional Health Practitioners Bill, was passed into law. Yet the potentiality of T&CM integration into the health system remains largely unfulfilled, unlike in Ghana there is no national policy on regulating the use of traditional plant-based medicines in Kenya (Gakuya et al:2020).

Beyond the Ghanaian and Kenyan context, evidence for the successful integration of T&CM within African health care systems remains relatively sparse with the exception of South Africa. Here the integration of traditional health practitioners (THPs) has been much more systematic than in either Ghana or Kenya. The total number of THPs in the country is estimated to be over 300,000, this equates to a population ratio of more than 1:170 (Flint & Payne:2013). In 2007, the South African government introduced its *Traditional Health Practitioners* (THP) *Act 22*. The objective of this legislation was to formalise and professionalise the practice of TPHs so as to enable their collaboration with biomedical professionals to jointly provide primary health care services. This development was overtly presented as consistent with the government principle of 'decolonialising medicine' and removing its associations with the authority of the former colonial power. A decade after the implementation of the THP legislation, one evaluative study concluded that, 'THP's have successfully been integrated into biomedical programmes after undergoing training in HIV prevention strategies, and used to train other practitioners .... (therefore) clinical traditional practitioner-biomedical co-operation is therefore practicable' (de Roubaix:2016;159). According to the study's authors, many patients now regard biomedicine and traditional medicine as equally important in South Africa and visit both THPs and biomedical clinics before starting on HIV/Aids anti-retroviral treatment.

The introduction of the traditional practitioners legislative framework in South Africa has undoubtedly played a significant role in their integration into the health care system. However, it has also been said that the legislation was simply a formal recognition of what already existed on the ground given that it has been estimated that up to 80% of black South Africans rely on THPs for health care. Whether this is through personal choice or out of necessity due to limited access to, mainstream medical services is unclear (de Roubaix:2016;160). What can be said is that the strategy has been as much about pragmatism as fulfilling the principle of integration. Facilitating a system of THPs does not compensate for the failure to construct an efficient and comprehensive medical care service for the whole population. Here there are clear similarities with the Ghanaian experience, particularly in those rural regions of the country where investment both in the state and private health care service sectors has historically failed to meet rising local health needs.

****

A comparative outcomes analysis of the Ghanaian and Kenyan health systems

The comparative analysis of the Ghanaian and Kenyan health systems set out in the following section utilises an assessment framework consisting of six evaluative outcome categories, each with an associated set of descriptors. The six categories reflect performance criterion that can in principle be applied to the assessment of any health care system, but the descriptors for each evaluative category do reflect the particular challenges faced by LIDC health systems.[12] Each of the descriptors, their outcome measures and their data sources are described under their respective evaluative category heading below; noting that the evaluative categories and their descriptors are represented in schematic form in Chapter 5, Table 5.3.

Note: An important consideration in attempting to compare the performance outcomes of health systems in Sub-Saharan Africa is, with some exceptions, the relative paucity of health data. This situation has improved in recent years with the roll-out of networked health information systems (HISs) in both Ghana and Kenya. But limitations remain in terms of the range and availability of up-to-date information and this can make it challenging to fully assess each of the descriptors of system outcome performance. Nevertheless, many of the countries in the African region are committed to making progress on the UN SDGs and the long-term goal of UHC, so that the production of 'routine' and reliable health information is a priority.

1. Quality and delivery of services
Health service availability and readiness
The data used to evaluate this descriptor derives from a WHO monitoring survey known as the 'Service Availability and Readiness Assessment' (SARA). The survey is a based on a methodology developed through a joint WHO and United States Agency for International Development (USAID) collaboration, and designed 'to fill critical gaps in measuring and tracking progress in health systems strengthening, (and to) support national planners in managing health systems' (WHO:2015;9). The survey relies on data supplied by key informants interviewed in the field, combined with national health system and census data, 'undertaken under the overall leadership of a country's Ministry of Health' (WHO:2015;10). The package of health services in a national health system assessed by a SARA survey for the purposes of assessing 'service availability' primarily focuses on the density of the health workforce, hospitals and clinics expressed as a per head of population ratio. The service 'readiness' component of SARA is assessed on the basis of five domains: basic amenities, basic equipment, standard precautions for infection prevention, diagnostic capacity, and essential medicines. The overall health service availability and readiness for a particular health system is assessed on the basis of the total capacity of a range of primary, preventive, and secondary health care services. Altogether over 500 aspects of specific health service capacity are measured in a SARA survey for a given health system (WHO:2015;128). It should be noted that the SARA survey does not directly generate data on either the quality or affordability of health services, but it does assess whether the infrastructural preconditions for developing high-quality and affordable services exist in a particular health system.

In 2019, the last available data point, the overall SARA index score for Ghana was 47% and for Kenya it was 55% (WHO Regional Office for Africa:2023a). To provide some context, Kenya was slightly above, and Ghana at the median of SARA scores for those Sub-Saharan countries where data was available. One of the several ways in which the WHO Regional Office for Africa (AFRO) monitors the pathway to UHC the respective is the 'average coverage of essential services amongst the general population', in 2019 the scores were 45% in Ghana and 56% in Kenya; the median score in the WHO AFRO

Region was 46%. The respective scores in 2019 for the reproductive, maternal, and child health services availability component of UHC, which is calculated as the geometric mean of family planning, antenatal care visits, childhood immunisation, and suspected pneumonia, was 68 for Ghana and 73 for Kenya; the median score for the WHO AFRO Region being 55 (WHO Regional Office for Africa:2022).

Meeting international disease management standards and regulations

The data used to assess comparative performance in relation to this evaluative descriptor is derived from the disease treatment 'best practice' guidelines and standards broadly aligned with WHO recommendations. The outcome data is produced in both countries with the technical assistance of WHO AFRO Region consultants. Disease management standards are published and regularly updated by both the Ghanaian and Kenyan Ministries of Health (Ghana MoH:2017/Kenya MoH:2023). Alongside this data source is the evidence of trends in disease-reduction in both countries. The latter is a broad indication that the national guidelines are being implemented in the field. Assessment data comes in the form an individual country's International Health Regulations (IHR) capacity score.

The IHR is an instrument of international law that is legally binding on the 194 WHO member countries. These regulations were first adopted by the WHO in 1969 and initially covered just six diseases. Since that time these regulations have been revised and expanded in response to the expansion of international travel and trade, and the emergence, re-emergence, and international spread of disease and other threats to public health. The current regulations were adopted the 58th World Health Assembly on 2005 (WHO:2005), and 'provide an overarching legal framework that defines countries rights and obligations in handling public health events and emergencies that have the potential to cross borders' (WHO:2023b). The IHRs require that all countries have the ability to (a) 'detect': defined as ensuring surveillance systems and laboratories can detect potential threats, (b) 'assess': defined as working together with other countries to make joint decisions concerning public health emergencies, (c) 'report': defined as the requirement to report specific diseases, plus any potential international public health emergencies, through participation in a network of National Focal Points, and (d) 'respond': defined as pertaining to public health events (WHO:2005). An individual country's compliance with the international regulations on disease control is self-assessed annually, and scored according to its performance vis-à-vis the IHR 15 'core capacities' (assessed by 35 indicators). The 15 core capacities include (i) policy, legislation, and normative instruments, (ii) IHR coordination and National Focal Point functions, (iii) financing, (iv) laboratory capability, (v) disease surveillance, (vi) human resources, (vii) National Health Emergency Framework, (viii) Health Service Provision, (ix) infection prevention and control, (x) risk communication, (xi) point of entry into a country, (xii) zoonotic events, (xiii) food safety, (xiv) chemical events, and (xv) radiation emergencies (WHO:2021b;11).

The IHR 15 core capacity compliance score provided for Kenya in 2023 was 54%, and for Ghana it was 56%, this was above the median score for the WHO African Region that stood at 50% (WHO:2024a). Both countries improved on their IHR compliance scores from 2022, but it is difficult to be precise about the long-term improvement trend. This is because the IHR only widened to 15 core capacities in 2021, up from the previous 13 core capacities using 24 indicators.

Both the Ghanaian and Kenyan Ministries of Health point to improvements in disease management performance over the last decade. So for example, the most recent annual performance review produced by the Kenyan Ministry of Health reports a year-on-year increase in expenditure for specialised health services programmes. These monies are designated for the implementation of disease management guidelines and regulations. This annual review also included examples of 'best practice and innovation' in the quality assessment and efficiency at Kenyan regional health institutional levels (Kenya MoH:2022).

Implementation of international patient safety and quality assurance standards

The information and data used to assess performance in relation to this particular descriptor is primarily derived from the 'Atlas of African Health Statistics' (WHO Regional Office for Africa:2022). The WHO has estimated that some 60% of all deaths in health care services within low- and middle-income countries are attributable to poor quality care, and that this reflects a failure to implement basic international patient safety standards. The WHO African Region produces a data index for patient safety by country. This assessment tool includes scores based on health service institutional safety norms as well as the application of organisational guidelines. In 2022, this patient safety index gave Ghana a 'high score' of over 60%, while Kenya was given a 'low' score of below 40%; the average score for the WHO African Region as a whole was 61% (WHO Regional Office for Africa:2022;156).

Ghana did not develop a national patient safety strategy of its own until 2021, this was funded with the support of the European Union and aligned with the most recent WHO Global Patient Safety Action Plan (WHO:2021a). This strategy was developed following the outcome of a situational analysis conduced in 27 health facilities across the nine regions of Ghana (WHO Ghana:2022;20).

Kenya was one of the first countries in the African Region to conduct a national survey of patient safety in 2012. This survey found that just 2% of health facilities in Kenya were compliant with the minimum patient safety and quality assurance protocols recommended by the WHO at the time. The Ministry of Health report that reviewed these survey results recommended the development of what it termed a 'Total Quality Management Framework' to be implemented across all health facilities in the country (Kenya MoH:2013;32). This objective was subsequently incorporated within the national strategic plan entitled 'Kenya Health Policy 2014–2030' (Kenya MoH:2014). The latter sets out a pathway for the achievement of Kenya's constitutional commitment to a long-term development agenda in line with the UN SDGs alongside the adaption of the WHO system building recommendations. A dedicated 'Quality model for Patient Safety' was enacted by the Ministry of Health in 2018 (Kenya MoH:2018).

2. Patient and population outcomes
Information systems: monitoring, evaluation, and timely dissemination of reliable data

A key requirement in the monitoring the outcomes of a health system, and by extension its performance, is the existence of a reliable and systematic tool for the collection and collation of health data. These tools are known as HISs. Today, HISs generally take the form of dedicated digital platforms that collate health data from across a national network and as such constitute a national 'data warehouse' (Koumamba et al:2021;237). Several African health systems including Ghana have begun to construct their own health data 'warehouses' utilising an open-source software known as the District Health Management Information System (DHMIS), this is a process that has in part been supported and funded by a number of international aid agencies. The DHMIS platform uses comprehensive open source software that can be customised to meet the particular needs of the different branches of the health service, and it enables data compiled from standardised tools to be uploaded remotely from the field, even if that data is paper-based or recorded using a tablet or mobile phone.

Since 2008, the Ghana Health service has implemented a sequence of HIS developments centred on the roll-out of a national cluster of DHMIS. By 2013, 170 out of 216 health districts within the country had activated the platform, constituting over 5,000 registered users. By 2016, the number of registered health service users had doubled to over 10,000 (Odei-Lartey et al:2020). Access to a DHMIS (the latest iteration of the software is termed DHIS2) is now potentially unlimited across the Ghana Health service and is now routinely used as an immunisation programme tracker to assess population coverage, for logistics planning, and for reporting the outbreak of disease epidemics. Nevertheless, the Internet connectivity upon which this digital platform crucially depends for its operation remains patchy outside the local state capital's. This creates challenges for the process of data synchronisation and completeness. Health workers in the field often have to travel to their local state capital in order to access the internet and then submit their data collection material onto the platform e-tracker (Nabunnya:2022). The point being that despite the clear functionality of this dedicated software, a truly effective HIS requires a national level of investment in digital infrastructures that is often beyond the fiscal means of many if not most LIDCs. On this last point, it is also noted that there are many parts of rural Europe where an effective digital infrastructure is still to be constructed.

The Kenyan Ministry of Health has also more recently been engaged in the development of what it describes as a 'robust' HIS. This system when fully rolled-out will be essential for collating standardised performance indicator data that can effectively track the progress being made (or not as the case maybe) towards meeting Kenya's commitment to achieving the 2030 SDG goals, and progressing its 'Kenya Health Policy 2014–2030'. The e-infrastructure required for the construct and effective operation of this digital platform was outlined in the Ministry of Health's 'Monitoring and Evaluation Plan 2018–2030' (Kenya MoH:2019). Yet a key feature of any HIS is the functionality of its 'interoperability', defined as 'the capacity for different information systems to meaningfully exchange data … (to enable an HIS) to be implemented across organisational boundaries to effectively deliver healthcare services' (Nyangena et al:2021;3). It is difficult to precisely assess the current effective functionality and readiness of the Kenyan HIS, but independent peer-reviewed research conducted in 2021 which assessed three key domains of Kenya's HIS interoperability framework (leadership and governance, human resources, and technology), concluded that, '(N)one of these domains had a maturity level greater than level 2' (Nyangena et al:2021;1). Level 2 (emerging) is the second lowest on a 5-level scale of system maturity. Level 2 is designated as a country having 'defined health information structures (HIS) but they are not systematically documented. No formal or ongoing monitoring or measurement protocol exits'. By contrast, level 5 maturity of a HIS is defined as 'optimised', where 'government and stakeholders routinely review interoperability activities and modify them to adapt to changing conditions' (Nyangena et al:2021;3).

Population coverage of public health programmes

In January 2017, at the 28th African Union (AU) Summit, Heads of State from across Africa endorsed what has subsequently become known as the 'Addis Declaration on Immunization' (ADI). This declaration committed the member countries to increase their political, financial, and technical investments in public health programmes in order to accelerate progress towards achieving universal access to immunisation, a key precondition for meeting many of the UN SDGs. Despite the significant early progress that had been made in increasing access to immunisation programmes for communicable diseases, with some now on the brink of eradication such as polio and neo-natal tetanus, national and subnational immunisation coverage rates have stagnated in many African countries over the past two decades: 'The African Region still lags behind other regions of the world in access to vaccines. Approximately 1 in 5 African children do not receive all the necessary and basic vaccines. As a result, more than 30 million children under five still suffer from vaccine-preventable diseases (VPDs) every year in Africa' (WHO Regional Office for Africa:2023b).

In 2021, the Ghanaian and Kenyan health systems respectively achieved an 89% and 91% measles immunisation coverage, and in relation to polio immunisation, 98% and 94% respectively in their populations. In the same year, the WHO African Region had the lowest global vaccination rate amongst one-year olds for DTP3 (Diphtheria, tetanus toxoid, and pertussis) equating to a 72% coverage (WHO Regional Office for Africa:2022;23). However, both Ghana and Kenya achieved a much higher rate of DTP3 immunisation cover for children under the age of one at 98% and 91% respectively. Additional to these immunisation programmes, family planning is another important component of public health programmes, particularly as they have the potential to contribute to meeting a wide range of SDG objectives. These include a reduction in child mortality, improving maternal health, as well as promoting women's empowerment and gender equality so enabling wider participation in school, work, and political life. In the WHO African Region, 79% of the primary health facilities offer family planning services, yet 'there remains high variability across countries in meeting the goal for women of four or more antenatal visits, ranging from 32% to 91%' (WHO Regional Office for Africa:2022;164).

In meeting the WHO targets for antenatal care visits, Ghana achieved a 87% coverage rate in 2020, while Kenya saw just 58% of pregnant women receiving antenatal visits in the same year. Maternal mortality rates have been steadily falling in Ghana over the past decade, and in 2020 stood at 176 (per 100,000 live births). Over the same period, Kenya also initially saw a slight reduction in rates, but since 2017 the numbers have climbed significantly to a rate of 530 maternal deaths per 100,000 live births in 2020 (iAHO:2023). The Kenyan Ministry of Health Performance Review 2020/21 does not acknowledge these WHO statistics, instead it has chosen to publish data that focuses only on maternal deaths within but not outside of formal health facilities. This is a quite separate measure known as the Faculty Maternal Mortality Rate (FMMR), and has remained constant in Kenya since 2015. This Ministry of Health performance review does however acknowledge that: '(T)he FMMR may not be accurate in depicting which counties had the highest maternal deaths as more deaths may take place in the community for counties with low skilled birth coverage' (Kenya MoH:2022;83). This comment is an implicit acknowledgement of the uneven level of health provision across the country, so that mothers living in the poorer rural areas (counties) of the country generally experience much higher rates of mortality due to limited availability of efficient maternal services.

Social differences in morbidity and mortality rates

Social epidemiologists have long understood that significant differences in health outcomes (typically measured by mortality and morbidity rates) exist between socioeconomic classes. This outcome is recognised as reflecting lifelong differences in material living standards and social and educational life chances.[13] However, it is only relatively recently that social differences in health outcome were given due prominence in research studies of health outcomes in African countries. There has been an unfortunate tendency, even in the recent past, to homogenise the health and life chances of African populations, as if low average per capita incomes somehow apply to all who live and work in these countries rather than being what it actually is, a statistical average. In practice, the socio-economic gap in health outcomes that exist within populations across the Sub-Saharan African region are as proportionately wide, if not wider than in HICs.

The UN utilises what it terms the 'human development index' (HDI) to monitor national progress towards the implementation of the 2030 Agenda for Sustainable Development (UN:2015). HDI is a composite index based on three indicators: life expectancy, education, and income. Some has been made in several African countries in improving health and life chances over the past two decades, as measured by an increase in their HDI score; '(I)n particular thanks to the progress in access to drinking water, sanitation, and hygiene. But the progress made could be reversed if efforts are not made to face the threats linked to climate change and inequalities' (WHO Regional Office for Africa:2022;11). This reinforces the point that public health measures alone will not significantly reduce the social gap in health outcomes within these same countries.

One of the key indicators of a country's progress towards meeting UN SDG 3 (Good Health and Well-being) is the trend in rates of mortality (life-expectancy) and morbidity (disease). Over the period of two decades, from 2000 to 2019, both Ghana and Kenya have seen a similar increase in life expectancy at birth, in the former, from 59 to 66 years, and in the latter from 54 to 66 years. This may or may not be linked to improvements in the overall standard of living in these countries, but again it is a statistical average and does not examine differences in life expectancy between social classes. Utilising a rather less crude measure known as 'healthy life expectancy at birth' (the average number of years that a person can expect to live in 'full health' by taking into account years lived in less than full health due to disease and/or injury – WHO:2023a), the improvement in life expectancy in both Ghana and Kenya appears to be rather less impressive. Ghana has seen an increase in healthy life expectancy from 52 years to 58 over the same two decades, while in Kenya it has increased from 47 to 58 years. As a comparator, the average healthy life expectancy found across the WHO

Europe Region in 2019 was 68.3 years (WHO Europe:2022). Healthy life expectancy outcomes necessarily involve social, political, and economic interventions that go well beyond the remit of any given health care system.

3. Equity and sustainability
Distributive justice: how are the benefits and costs of health care distributed?

A key statistic, albeit a crude one, in assessing a government's commitment to delivering on health equity and the achievement of UHC, is the percentage of the national budget that is allocated to overall health spending. When Organisation of African Union member states met in Abuja, Nigeria in 2001, over two decades ago, to address the epidemics of HIV/Aids, Tuberculosis, and other infectious disease then rampant across the continent, each member government agreed to commit 15% of annual state spending to health from that point forward. This commitment became known as the Abuja Declaration (OAU:2001). However, in the years following this declaration; 'government spending on health, as a proportion of its overall spending, *decreased* in 21 African countries between 2001 and 2015. Development assistance for health has crowded out government resources and created donor dependence' (Gatome-Munyua & Olalere:2020).

In 2022, health spending by the state in Ghana represented just 7.6% of the government total spending budget. While for the Kenyan Government, the equivalent figure was just 8.0% (WHO Regional Office for Africa:2022). In short, both governments are currently committing just about half the amount that they signed up to just over 20 years ago. This state of affairs is as much a reflection of the continuing weakness of their respective economies as it is the impact of competing priorities for government resources. An additional factor in play is the failure in both countries to develop an efficient and fair system of state revenue collection. This does reflect the fact that the majority of the working population are in the informal sector of the economy which in turn makes it difficult to assess and collect income tax, and so a reliance is placed on regressive consumption taxes. The result is that in both countries, the benefits and costs of health care are unevenly distributed as between socio-economic classes, and between rural and urban areas. This outcome is reflected in the disproportionate reliance on regressive OOPs for health care costs by the majority of those with lower incomes in both countries.

In 2022, the United Nations International Children's Emergency Fund published its first wave country-level and WHO regional-level data in a publication entitled 'Countdown to 2030' (UNICEF:2023). This charts global progress towards the meeting of the 2030 SDGs and includes a range of indicators of individual country's population coverage for RMNCAH (reproductive, maternal, newborn, child and adolescent health) primary care interventions and associated immunisation programmes. The key indicator of a country's progress in widening coverage is its 'Equity profile'. This is assessed using several measures that include educational level, socio-economic status, gender, age, and place of residence (rural or urban). UNICEF also provides a single numerical measure of equity in relation to RMNCAH coverage for each country, this is known as the 'composite coverage index' (CCI).[14] Figure 6.3 provides a CCI percentage figure for RMNCAH equity in Kenya and Ghana, assessed by socio-economic status using the proxy measure of income quintiles (the population is separated into five bands, with Q1 being the poorest 20% and Q5 the richest 20%).

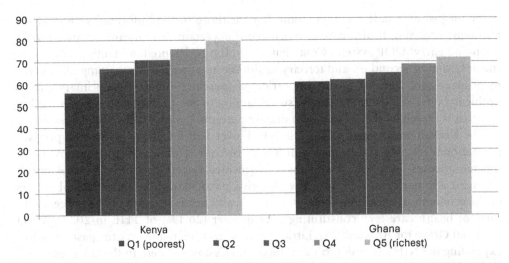

Figure 6.3 Kenya and Ghana – RMNCAH equity profile composite coverage index (CCI) by socio-economic status (Adapted from iAHO (2023)).

Figure 6.3 demonstrates that RMNCAH service coverage is not equitable in both Kenya and Ghana, but the socio-economic divide is wider in the former. While the proportion of GDP spent in both countries is broadly comparable, using the CCI measure of RMNCAH coverage by socio-economic status, it is possible to say that health spending in Ghana is more equitably distributed across the population. In recent years, both health systems have attempted to address regional disparities in the provision of health resource through a strategy of decentralisation. However, balancing-up regional inequities in health provision does not mean that the 'national pie', the annual health spending budget, has become larger. Addressing social inequities in health service provision requires a much more deliberative health policy approach.

Health system financing: cost-risk pooling and the role of public and private insurance funding

Cost-risk pooling ensures that the financial burden associated with an individual funding their family's health care needs is ameliorated through collective contributions, transferred to some form of health care purchasing organisation.[15] The existence of the pool enables a transfer of funds or cross-subsidy to be made from those with a low health risk to those at high risk. Meeting the objective of UHC in a given country requires the widest possible pooling of financial risk becomes a primary policy objective. In this process, the state necessarily must play an active interventionary role, it cannot be left to the unregulated private market (Mathauer et al:2019;1).

Government expenditure as a percentage of THE in both Kenya and Ghana is around the 50% mark (see Figure 6.2). However, the process of cost-risk pooling has advanced further in Ghana than Kenya. Though the NHIS established by the Ghanaian government in 2003 is not a compulsory scheme it is potentially open to all citizens and their families. As discussed earlier in this chapter, the NHIS currently provides health risk cover for just over half the population, but for those in the 'informal' sectors of the economy, accessing health care is much more uncertain, and means reliance on the 'cash-and-carry' OOP system. Contributions to the NHIS predominantly (80%) go to the provision of secondary and tertiary health services, with the remaining 20% going to primary care services. Small proportion of spending allocated to primary care is problematic for the overall financial sustainability of the health service, given the key role that is played by these services in disease prevention and healthy life promotion.

The Kenyan government set up the NIHF over half-a-century ago as the primary institutional form of risk-pooled health care revenue. Despite several reforms to the scheme since its inception, it remains a fragmented system that only provides health cover for a minority of Kenyans. The majority, particularly those in informal sectors of the economy, are required to pay for their health needs through OOPs, a regressive form of health care levy constituting over quarter (26.1%) of THE in 2022 (WHO Regional Office for Africa:2022). Little progress has been made over the past decade in expanding the NIHF in order to meet the country's commitment to the achievement of UHC by 2030, the central plank of 'The Kenya Plan 2014–30' (see above).

4. Governance and accountability
Health system capacity for reform and quality improvement

Both Kenya and Ghana are committed in principle to the decentralisation of the health resource allocation decision-making process so that it becomes the prerogative of regional authorities. In Ghana's case, this process began several decades ago and is more accurately described as 'deconcentration', where authority moves to regional institutions but that they remain accountable to the central Ministry of Health. In Kenya, following the constitutional reforms of 2010, decentralisation is closer to the ideal of regional 'devolution'. The distinction drawn between these forms of decentralisation follows Rondeinelli's (1981) typology of decentralisation in LIDCs (cited in Rodríguez et al:2023;632). The objective of both strategies of decentralisation is to promote regional governance so that the health system is more reactive and responsive to local health needs. Yet this ideal has been stymied in both countries by the failure to restructure the levers of bureaucratic centralised control, as exercised by the respective Ministries of Health. In both countries, there has been a general failure to build into the process any substantive governance mechanisms that mandate meaningful community engagement.

At the very least, a publicly accountable system of health governance requires transparent access to valid and reliable performance data. Both the Kenyan and Ghanaian Ministries of Health, in collaboration with the WHO African Region, regularly publish reports on the performance of key health sector indicators. But this performance data is often less than comprehensive and not always contemporaneous. This in turn raises questions about the utility of each country's recently developed HISs, and the continuing reliance on paper-based information systems. The Kenyan Ministry of Health had produced publicly available annual performance reviews for nearly two decades, although their appearance has been somewhat sporadic. As of late 2024, the last available performance review was published in October 2022 for the financial year 2020–21 (Kenya MoH:2022). In Ghana, the national statistical service (GSS) has for over a decade produced *The Health Sector in Ghana Facts and Figures,* an annual report on the performance of selected health sector indicators. But Ghana, like Kenya, does not have a fully developed Health Service Performance Assessment tool (HSPA), although it currently is in the process of developing one (Kumah et al:2021;3).

The WHO defines an HSPA as being balanced in scope and able to gather information about the functioning of the whole health system, not limited to specific programmes. The recommendation is that this information then should inform policy decisions, monitor subsequent interventions, and as such, constitutes a key mechanism of governance (Papanicolas et al:2022). The rolling-out of the District Management Information System (DHMIS) in both health systems is described above, but however valuable it is as data collection tool, a DHMIS does not constitute an HSPA. The concern here is that robust systems of governance should include transparent and accessible health system performance data, reliance on an HIS where only selected policy actors have access is not an alternative. This is particularly the case when the use of a HIS is fragmented between the needs of local health care teams and external donor agencies. The latter tend to require the collection of health data that meet the objectives of their own health programmes, but who 'have little involvement in more comprehensive strategies for developing and managing more integrated HIS' (Koumamba et al:2021;238).

Implementation and enforcement of regulatory frameworks across all system activities

In the context of their analysis of the Kenyan health care system, Oraro-Lawrence and Wyss have posed the rhetorical question, 'what constitutes an effective system of health care governance?' Their answer was that such a system should be able to; 'focus on defining a common and realistic set of health system values, as well as creating a strong policy, legal, institutional and regulatory framework to support the progressive achievement of UHC' (2020;9). Rather than attempting to provide a fully comprehensive analysis of the full range of regulatory mechanisms in operation in both health systems, this section will examine the regulation of medical professional practice as a case study of the relative efficacy of the existing structures of governance.

In Ghana, the legal framework of professional regulation is defined in law by the 2013 Health Professions Regulatory Bodies Act. This legislation established separate regulatory councils for the Allied Health Professionals, Doctors and Dentists, Nurses and Midwives, Pharmacists, and Psychologists. Specifically, in relation to the medical profession, this legislation established the Medical and Dental Council (essentially the equivalent of the General Medical Council in the UK) charging the Council with the legal responsibility for enforcing professional standards, having oversight of professional training and qualifications, and managing the professional register. The Ghanaian Medical Council has stated that its 'vision' for the role of the Council was as, 'an accountable regulatory authority for medical and dental practice in Ghana for the public good' (Medical and Dental Council of Ghana:2023). Yet specifics about the regulatory mechanisms designed to ensure patient safety and public accountability do not appear in the legal mandate that established the Medical Council. Its governing body consists of 11 members, of which only two are lay members; it is therefore essentially a self-regulatory body. The lessons that were painfully learnt in the UK and in other HIC health systems concerning the necessity of having a formal set of regulatory requirements that legally ensure that medical professionals are held publicly accountable for their practise does not seem to have been learnt.[16]

There is a distinct paucity of research that has examined the efficacy of the system of medical professional governance in both countries. But one recent qualitative research study carried out in Kenya and neighbouring Uganda, reported that both doctors and nurses would welcome good regulatory relations, and while they felt that the existing regulatory standards in both countries were 'appropriate' they were seen to be 'poorly implemented'. The professional regulatory bodies in both countries were described as lacking both the financial and the human resources to function effectively; 'Doctors and nurses generally described limited relations and interactions with "remote" regulators, who were seen to be more interested in collecting fees than regulating professional practice' (McGivern et al:2021;2). The participants in the study also criticised their own professional regulatory councils as frequently too lenient on colleagues found to be negligent or having engaged in malpractice. Criticism was also levelled at the failure of the regulatory councils 'to better communicate and improve professionals own understanding of what regulation and standards mean in practice ... regulators can further enhance the social accountability of professionals by making it clearer and easier to report such malpractice' (McGivern et al:2021;7). The recommendation of this report was for systems of professional regulation to be decentralised, so that professionals could work with local regulators to address local problems. However, the study also reported a concern that local level politics could then interfere with effective local regulatory processes (McGivern et al:2021;8). In summary, decentralisation alone is not an unproblematic 'solution' to the problem of ineffective centralised systems of health governance.

5. Efficiency
Allocative efficiency

Allocative efficiency refers to the distribution of resources across an entire sector of health care interventions.[17] In LIDC health systems, including those of Kenya and Ghana, limited health resources must be fully optimised in order to meet health system goals. But as previously discussed, given the relative underdevelopment of the HISs of both countries there is only a limited range of data available to measure allocative efficiency. As a consequence undue reliance is placed on less than specific epidemiological data such as national mortality and morbidity statistics in order to direct resources to where they are deemed to have most benefit (WHO Regional Office for Africa:2022;136).

In Mbau et al's (2023) recent systematic review, it is clear that allocative efficiency is impacted not only by internal institutional resource issues, but also by factors 'exogenous' to that system. These factors are seen to include: '(T)he demographic and socio-economic characteristics of the population, macro-economic characteristics of the national and sub-national regions, population health and well-being, the governance and political characteristics of these regions, and health system characteristics' (Mbau et al:2023;206). It is for this reason that the authors state that it is challenging to summarise or compare efficiency findings across health systems given the heterogeneity of the methods that are used. On this point, it is noteworthy that the most recent WHO statistical atlas does not provide any definitive overarching efficiency ranking for African health systems (WHO Regional Office for Africa:2022). This systematic review goes on to cite an efficiency analysis of 141 countries conducted by the WHO which found that the relative rankings were highly sensitive to the definition of efficiency that was employed and to the choice of assessment model (Mbau et al:2023;214). The authors concluded that a distinction should be drawn between analyses that assess the performance of a health system as a whole and those that are focused on distinct system outputs. The latter is the approach that is adopted in the comparative assessment framework utilised in this chapter.

Technical efficiency of health system

The reductive basis on which technical efficiency analyses is generally conducted is that systems must manage their resources to maximise every pound and penny spent on health care provision. A recent technical efficiency analysis of 36 African health care systems expands on this 'data-driven' process: 'Although the healthcare system of each country is unique due to countries' historical and socioeconomic differences, all healthcare systems have functions such as providing accessible and effective health services to individuals at an optimum cost' (Top et al:2020;62). Similarly, a recent report published by the WHO African Region, entitled *Technical efficiency of health systems in the WHO African Region*, noted that: '(I)mproving efficiency of health systems calls for actions beyond health financing alone ... (these include) addressing fragmentations and duplications in the different building blocks of the system; strengthening management; addressing gaps in quality of care; rationalization of health infrastructure expansion to improve access and utilization of services; embracing use of digital technologies; and ensuring equitable availability of skilled workforce' (WHO Regional Office for Africa:2023c;viii).

Both of these comparative technical efficiency studies employ a methodology known as 'data envelopment analytical' (DEA). DEA scores are calculated according to best practice and are bounded between 0 and 1. This process is said to allow for multiple inputs with different denominators and trends, and so it is 'more appropriate for measuring the technical efficiencies' of African health systems (WHO Regional Office for Africa:2023c;8). It is useful to provide some further explanatory detail regarding the methodology of DEA, given the generally acknowledged complexity of assessing the technical efficiency of health systems.[18] There are four main stages in the process. Firstly, a systematic review of the empirical literature is conducted, this then informs a narrative analysis that generates the selection of which input and output efficiency variables will be chosen. Secondly, a 'cross-programmatic' efficiency analysis is conducted consisting of qualitative synthesis reports for a specific health system, this is used to identify potential allocative efficiency gains. The third stage is to conduct the DEA itself using a statistical regression analysis of the identified drivers of efficiency. Finally, an 'integrative meta-synthesis' is carried out, this synthesises the findings from the three previous stages into one composite report that describes 'the efficiency, drivers and potential areas of policy actions' (WHO Regional Office for Africa:2023c;5).

The main findings of the WHO African Region technical efficiency report were that the majority of countries in the region were operating at 80% levels of efficiency in the period of 2019, which by extension meant that they were operating at a 20% level of inefficiency. In financial terms, this inefficiency equated to some US$30 billion across the region. Nevertheless, this efficiency rating did represent a significant improvement on an analysis conducted five years previously in 2014, when only an average 67% technical efficiency rating was recorded. The report concluded that, 'improving technical efficiency alone will yield a maximum of 34% improvement in resource availability in African health systems – assuming all countries are performing at a similar level. However, with the low level of health expenditure per capita in Africa, the efficiency gains alone will likely be insufficient to meet the maximum requirement for Universal

Health Coverage' (WHO Regional Office for Africa:2023c;32). This conclusion follows because if the technical efficiency of the *existing* structures of health care can be maximised, this will still only bring about a finite improvement. What is required to meet the requirements of UHC necessitates addressing the 'fragmentations and duplications in the different building blocks of the health system', an improvement in the quality of care, and a rationalisation of the infrastructure of health care (WHO Regional Office for Africa:2023c;32).

The WHO African Region technical efficiency rating for the Ghanaian health system was 64%, well below the regional average, equating to a loss of US$26.85 per capita (current per capita expenditure being US$75.28). In the case of Kenya, there was insufficient input and output data available in order to be able to arrive at an equivalent technical efficiency score. However, based on the average scores of five independent studies previously conducted using the DEA methodology, Kenya was deemed to have a systems level efficiency score of around 85% (WHO Regional Office for Africa:2023c;16). A more recent efficiency study of the Kenyan system, utilising a qualitative cross-sectional methodology, focused on the impact of the policy of decentralisation on technical efficiency. It concluded that, 'duplication, fragmentation, and misalignment of health system functions and actor actions compromise the coordination of the health sector in Kenya' (Nyawira et al:2023;1).

6. Access and responsiveness
Accessibility of health services
The data drawn upon to assess this indicator of health system performance derives from the WHO AFRO Country Health Systems and Services Profile – CHSSP (iAHO:2023). This source provides data on health facility, health worker, and hospital bed density scores (see also the 'service availability' section above). Kenya has a 'health facility density' of 1.41 per 100,000 population, while Ghana a density of 1.30. But these numbers only provide a partial picture of accessibility, they do not into take account the inequitable distribution of facilities and staff as between urban and rural areas. Nor do density scores reflect the geographical accessibility and travel time to health facilities. For example, a recent study of women who gave birth in the Eastern Region of Ghana found that it required more than two hours of travel time to attend maternal health services this resulted in a marked decrease in the utilisation of these services (Dotse-Gborgbortsi et al:2023). Density ratios also say little about the quality of the training and skills of the workforce who deliver care within these health facilities. In the historical-institutional outline of the Ghanaian and Kenyan and health systems set out in the first part of this chapter, it was noted that health facilities were concentrated in the main cities, and in particular the respective capitals, Accra and Nairobi. The cities have proportionally more hospitals per head of population, better equipped, and a higher than national average medical staff to patient ratios, and who are also often better trained and more experienced than staff in the rural and provincial regions.

Numbers of trained health care staff have expanded in both countries over the past two decades, but both systems continue to have density rates below the recommended WHO SDG threshold of 4.45 health workers per 1,000 population. Many of the factors that are complicit in the failure to develop the workforce in order to meet rising health demand have been discussed above, but include rapid population growth, inadequate training capacity, push-pull migration, poor retention, and the limited fiscal and political capacity of the state to grow the public health care sector (Ahmat et al:2022).

Integrated health care services: example – the management of childhood illnesses

Integrating patient care services can be a positive example of sustainable practice within a system, serving to optimise service utilisation and therefore efficient use of health resources, improvements in the patient experience (see below), and a reduction in health inequalities. The integration of health services can occur at different levels, horizontally across primary and secondary care settings, as well as vertically within a single institutional structure, resulting at least in theory, in improvements in clinical communication and information-sharing. This section will examine one example of system care integration, the integrated management of childhood illness (IMCI), as it has been implemented within the Ghanaian and Kenyan health systems.

The WHO and UNICEF jointly developed a global IMCI strategy with the aim of improving health worker skills, health service provision, as well as preventative practices for childhood illness within primary care and local communities. By the mid-1990s, over 100 countries had adopted and began the process of implementing the strategy. A Cochrane review found that the IMCI strategy was associated with a 15% reduction in child mortality when activities were implemented at scale in health facilities and communities (Gera et al:2012). Signing-up to this strategy requires the national adoption of IMCI standards, as well as ensuring the regular review of IMCI protocols adapted to a specific country's childhood disease epidemiology, and health system provision. In the African context, the ideal-type IMCI strategy would require: '(A) comprehensive assessment of a child's health status be undertaken and latent problems be detected, if possible, plus preventive interventions be provided such as vaccination and growth monitoring, and prevention or reduction of progression of diseases' (WHO Regional Office for Africa:2022;169). As noted by the WHO, in order to achieve SDG target 3.2 that specifies reducing child mortality to 25 or less deaths per 1,000 live births by 2030; 'it is paramount that key components of IMCI are implemented at scale, especially in countries with a high burden of preventable childhood mortality' (WHO:2024b).

The IMCI strategy was first adopted by the Ghanaian health system in 1999, but it was never systematically rolled out across the whole service: '(T)here have been no nationwide training efforts, no IMCI specific focal people at any level of the health system, and no large-scale partner support for many years. IMCI strategies are currently implemented in only 11 of Ghana's 216 districts. With 8.5% of Polyclinics providing the highest proportion of IMCI services, and just 1% of Community Health Planning Service[19] (CHPS) facilities' (Ghana Health Service:2023). Momentum, a partner agency that works with the national governments to implement global health programmes and interventions funded by the US Agency for International Development (USAID), recently produced an assessment report of the challenges to fully implementing IMCI within the Ghanaian health system (MOMENTUM:2023).

The report published by the Momentum Aid organisation acknowledges that while some elements of IMCI have been integrated into some specific child health programmes such as integrated supportive supervision checklists and malaria treatment protocols, it remains underdeveloped as a health strategy in Ghana due to the presence of four key barriers: (i) The under-resourcing of CHPS preventative services seen as peripheral within the Ghanaian health system since their inception, in large part due to the fact that they do not receive reimbursement from the NHIS. (ii) Over-reliance on international funding and international agency partner implementation whose goals are not always in alignment with Ghanaian national health priorities. (iii) Existing referral systems for IMCI were compromised by the lack of availability of transport for sick children and their caregivers. Overcoming this barrier was seen to require a review of ambulance availability throughout Ghana, especially in rural districts, and the consideration of alternative models, including community-supported transport initiatives. (iv) Widespread 'stock-outs' of medicines essential to IMCI service delivery. A shortage of essential medicines and equipment leading to unnecessary referrals, inappropriate OOP costs for caregivers, mistrust between caregivers and providers, and decreased morale for providers (MOMENTUM:2023;6). This report is also quite clear about the failings of the Ghana Health Service to develop the organisational and funding structures that are necessary to deliver on its own policy commitment to IMCI, 'as the most efficient and sustainable strategy for managing long-term child health' (MOMENTUM:2023;13).

While the barriers to establishing a health system-wide IMCI strategy in Ghana are considerable, the situation in Kenya is in many ways even more exacting. The implementation of the IMCI strategy has been government policy since 1999, but has consistently been under-resourced. A case study (Mullei et al:2008) has identified many inadequacies associated with implementation particularly in rural districts of the country. The report identified lack or limited coverage of IMCI training for health staff, medical stock-outs, and poor service infrastructure. The limitations of the NIHF that are discussed above manifest themselves as a key barrier to accessing IMCI services. This is particularly the case when children under five are charged user fees, where the lack of any health insurance cover can mean that the costs of referral (a key aspect of integrated child health care) result in a negative uptake and patient dropout from this service. One of the key recommendations of this case study is that District Health Management Teams (DHMT) should be given their own budgets to finance district-specific IMCI needs, including training and organisational provision for IMCI. This particular recommendation did finally come about following the 2012 health service decentralisation strategy.

A more recent survey of progress in implementing IMCI guidelines in Kenya has drawn on observational studies of health staff carrying out assessments of over 2000 sick children. It found that despite nationwide training for health staff in IMCI, adherence rates for assessment and physical examination protocols remained low and inconsistent, with staff consistently failing to recognise IMCI danger signs and primary symptoms (Krüger et al:2017). The recommendations of this study, were for further improvements in IMCI training, with particular emphasis on nurses, midwives, and auxiliary staff, to be 'consolidated with periodic re-training' (Krüger et al:2017;12).

In summary, the limited availability of health resources in both systems has resulted in significant gaps between 'aspirational' IMCI policies and the lack of effective service integration as between primary preventive and secondary health care providers. These limitations were combined with less than effective training programmes for health staff. This situation, particularly in the case of Kenya and to a lesser extent Ghana, is compounded by the fact that only a minority of the population are enrolled within a cost-risk pooled health insurance scheme, so remain reliant on OOPs for even their basic health needs. This leads to problems with patient retention, setting a further set of challenges for the integration of the management and care of childhood illness.

User experience

The reason that 'user experience' is included under this particular performance indicator is that unsatisfactory user experiences of the health service are likely to directly reflect issues associated with accessing even basic care provision, which remains a key issue in non-UHC systems (Titi-Ofei et al:2021).

The WHO Atlas of African Health Statistics (WHO Regional Office for Africa:2022) includes an index of 'user experience' by country. High satisfaction with the quality of health care service delivery generally occurs when health care providers exceed patient or user expectations in the delivery of services. The mean average index score across the WHO African Region was 54.9%, but this was top-and-tailed by two health systems that had scores exceeding 80%, and two systems with a user experience score below 20%. The user experience score for both Ghana and Kenya was relatively high for the region at over 70% (WHO Regional Office for Africa:2022;155). However, while the data sources of system performance are listed in the Atlas, there are no specifics concerning the methodology that was utilised to compile this comparative index of user satisfaction.

African societies, like all societies across the globe, are not homogenous, and differences in socio-economic class, place of residence, gender, as well as education level attained also play a key role in determining the health service user experience. This was the key finding of a Ghanaian study conducted by Amporfro et al (2021) that drew on data from the 2014 Ghana Demographic and Health survey that sampled nearly 13,000 households in order to assess the satisfaction of women patients with the provision of health services. This study chose to focus on the perspectives of women because in general they have been found to rely more on medical services than men, especially reproductive services. The study assessed three satisfaction-dependent variables (service reliability, service responsiveness, service tangibles), then the scores for each were combined together to produce a score for a fourth variable, 'total satisfaction'. The study found that high 'total' satisfaction scores (over 65%) were associated with younger women, women who lived in more affluent regions of Ghana, and those who had health insurance coverage as against using OOP to pay for services. There was also found to be a 'positive association' between higher levels of education and overall service satisfaction (Amporfro et al:2021;6–10).

Conclusions

In attempting to provide an over-arching evaluation of the developments that have occurred in both the Kenyan and Ghanaian health care systems since independence, institutional path-dependency theory has proven to be a constructive approach.[20] However, it cannot fully account for the contemporary formation and functioning of either system. The legacy of social exclusionary structures and uneven economic development in both these former British colonies have also been significant obstacles on the pathway to the building of robust inclusionary state structures, and that includes the health care system. However, in contradistinction to what is sometime referred to as the 'Afro-pessimism' school of thought,[21] an essentially lazy analysis that draws on crude stereotypes, the majority of African post-colonial states have proved themselves capable of building resilient health care structures. This is despite, not because of, the forced imposition of 'structural readjustment' programmes by the IMF and other global financial institutions in the 1980s. Yet the legacies of this neo-liberal economic approach continues to resonate in the constraints placed on national resources available to both finance and fund the national commitment to attaining UHC.

The evidence of the data presented under the six performance evaluative categories set out above, has demonstrated that there remain significant deficits in specific areas of provision in both health systems. But while being realistic about the continuing challenges faced in both Ghana and Kenya, progress has undoubtedly been made in constructing the infrastructure of a modern health care system in both countries.

Notes

1 The list of LDCs is reviewed every three years by the UN Committee for Development (CDP).
2 The impact of the IMF neo-liberal programmes of austerity on the development of the health care systems in both Ghana and Kenya is discussed in detail under each country heading set out below.
3 The collective name given to the four separate jurisdictions that constituted this British crown Colony in West Africa, from 1821 until independence in 1957.
4 Before becoming Prime Minister, Nkrumah was a renowned pan-Africanist and socialist, educated at the LSE in London, and later founder of the Organisation of African Unity (OAU) in 1962.
5 The epidemiological transition was first conceptualised by Abdel Omram in 1971. For Omran, this is a unidirectional process that moves from infectious diseases being the primary cause of death, manifested in high rates of childhood and maternal mortality, until significant improvements occur in the average standard of living, alongside effective public health interventions towards the end of the nineteenth century in Western Europe and North America. From this followed a 'transition' to chronic disease becoming the primary causes of mortality (Omran:1971).
6 Mental health service provision within the context of the UK is discussed in Chapter 9.
7 The challenge of providing health and social care to increasingly ageing populations in HICs is discussed in detail in Chapter 8.
8 According to Aiyar (2015), the brutal attack of the Westgate mall in Nairobi by the jihadist militant group, al-Shabaab, in September 2013 brought about a significant change in attitudes towards the East Asian community. The attack resulted in the death and injury of members of both East Asian and indigenous African communities. Asians were visibly involved in the rescue process as well as in the leading of vigils and other events in the wake of the attack, and this brought Kenyan citizens of different ethnic backgrounds together the banner of #WeAreOne on social media platforms.
9 'Germ Theory', following the work of Pasteur, Lister and later Koch, was consolidated by the late nineteenth century. This was the understanding that infectious disease causality involved the spread of microorganisms or pathogens into healthy tissues. However, it should be noted that the science of population disease epidemiology was only in its relative infancy by the start of the twentieth century.
10 This was post-colonial process that was identified as occurring in both former British and French territories by Frantz Fanon (1952/1967), described in his now classic 'Afro-pessimist' study, self-evidently entitled 'Black skins, White masks'.
11 Risk-pooling enables the higher costs of the less healthy to be offset by the relatively lower costs of the healthy – discussed in detail in Chapter 4.
12 The performance evaluative categories that constitute the basis of this framework for comparative health system analysis in LIDCs are described in detail in Chapter 5 and are represented in schematic form in Table 5.3 in the same chapter.
13 Social inequalities in health and their implications for the structuring of health policy interventions are discussed in Chapter 9.

14 UNICEF calculates CCI as, 'the weighted mean of eight selected interventions: demand for family planning; satisfied with modern methods; antenatal care (4+ visits); skilled birth attendant; care seeking for pneumonia; Oral rehydration salt solutions (ORS) for diarrhoea; and BCG, DTP3, and measles vaccines' (UNICEF:2023;29).

15 Cost-risk sharing and health care funding systems are described in detail in Chapter 4.

16 The process of regulating the medical profession in the UK is discussed in Chapter 3.

17 Described in detail in Chapter 5.

18 Described in Chapter 5.

19 The development of the CHPS is discussed in detail in the institutional account of the development of the Ghanaian health system in the first part of this chapter (Chapter 6).

20 Discussed in Chapter 2.

21 Outlined in the Introduction to Section III of this book.

References

Ahmat, A, Okoroafor, S, Kazanga, I, Asamani, J, Millogo, J, Illou, M, Mwinga, M and Nyoni, J (2022) The health workforce status in the WHO African Region: findings of a cross-sectional study, *BMJ Global Health*, vol. 7, e008317.

Aiyar, S (2015) *Indians in Kenya: The Politics of Diaspora*. Cambridge, Harvard. University Press.

Ampoefro, D, Boah, M, Yingqi, S, Wabo, T, Zhao, M, Nkondjock, V and Wu, Q (2021) Patient satisfaction with healthcare delivery in Ghana, *BMC Health Services Research*, vol. 21, no. 722, 1–13.

Barasa, E, Rogo, K, Mwaura, N and Chuma, J (2018) Kenya National Hospital insurance fund reforms: implications and lessons for universal health coverage, *Health Systems and Reform*, vol. 4, no. 4, 346–361.

Basu, S, Andrews, J, Kishore, S, Panjabi, R and Stuckler, D (2012) Comparative performance of private and public healthcare systems in low- and middle-income countries: a systematic review, *Public Library of Science (PLoS) Medicine*, vol. 9, no. 6, 1–13.

BBC News (2023) *Ghana patients in danger as nurses head for NHS in UK – medics*. June 6, 2023. https://www.bbc.co.uk/news/world-africa-65808660.

Christmals, C and Aidam, K (2020) Implementation of the National Health Insurance Scheme (NHIS) in Ghana: lessons for South Africa and low- and middle-income countries, *Risk Management and Health Care Policy*, vol. 13, 1879–1904.

Chuma, J and Okunga, V (2011) Viewing the Kenyan health system through an equity lens: implications for universal coverage, *International Journal for Equity in Health*, vol. 10, no. 22, 1–14.

de Roubaix, M (2016) The decolonialisation of medicine in South Africa: threat or opportunity? *South African Medical Journal*, vol. 106, no. 2, 159–161.

de-Graft Aikins, A and Koram, K (2017) 'Health and healthcare in Ghana, 1957–2017' in Aryeetey, E and Kanbur, R (eds) *The Economy of Ghana Sixty Years after Independence*. Oxford. Oxford University Press, pp 365–384.

Dotse-Gborgbortsi, W, Tatem, A, Matthews, Z, Alegana, V, Olosu, A and Wright, J (2023) Quality of maternal healthcare and travel time influence birthing service utilisation in Ghanaian health facilities: a geographical analysis of routine health data, *BMJ Open*, vol. 13, e066792.

Dovlo, D (2003) *The Brain Drain and the Retention of Health Professionals in Africa*. A case study prepared for a Regional Training Conference on Improving Tertiary Education in Sub-Saharan Africa: Things That Work! Accra, September 23–25, 2003. http://library.health.go.ug/.

Flint, A and Payne, J (2013) Reconciling the irreconcilable? HIV/AIDS and the potential for middle ground between the traditional and biomedical healthcare sectors in South Africa, *Forum for Development Studies*, vol. 40, no. 1, 47–68.

Gakuya, D, Okumu, M, Kiama, S, Mbaria, J, Gathumbi, P, Mathiu, P and Nguta, J (2020) Traditional medicine in Kenta: past and current status, challenges, and the way forward, *Scientific African*, vol. 8, e00360.

Gatome-Munyua, A and Olalere, N (2020) Public financing for health in Africa. *Africa Renewal*. October 2020. https://www.un.org/africarenewal/magazine.

Gera, T, Shah, D, Garner, P and Schdev, H (2012) Integrated management of childhood (IMCI) strategy for children under five: effects on death, service utilisation and illness, *Cochrane Database of Systematic Reviews*, no. 9.

Ghana Health Service (2023) *Innovative Solutions to Address Implementation and Resource Challenges in Integrated Management of Neonatal and Childhood Illness (IMNCI)*. https:// ghs.gov.gh (accessed 10/2023).

Ghana Ministry of Health (2017) *Standard Treat Guidelines* (7th Ed). Accra. MoH.

Ghana Statistical Service (2017) *Ghana Living Standards Survey, GLSS 7*. Accra. GSS.

iAHO – Integrated African Health Observatory WHO African Region (2023) *GPW13 Country Profiles*. https://aho.afro.who.int (accessed 01/2024).

International Monetary Fund (2019) *Macroeconomic Developments and Prospects in Low Income Developing Countries*. https://www.imf.org/external/pp/ppindex.aspx (accessed 10/ 2023).

International Monetary Fund [IMF] (1999) *The IMF's Enhanced Structural Adjustment Facility (ESAF): Is It Working?* https://www.imf.org/external/pubs/ft/esaf/exr/ (accessed 11/2022).

Kenya Ministry of Health (2014) *Kenya Health Policy 2014–2030*. Nairobi, Kenya. MoH. http:// publications.universalhealth2030.org/uploads/kenya_health_policy_2014_to_2030.pdf.

Kenya Ministry of Health (2018) *Core Standards for Quality Health Care: Kenya Quality Model for Health*. Nairobi, Kenya. Department of Health Standards, Quality Assurance and Regulation. MoH.

Kenya Ministry of Health (2019) *Kenya Health Sector Monitoring and Evaluation Plan*. Nairobi, Kenya. The Principal Secretary, Ministry of Health.

Kenya Ministry of Health (2022) *Health Sector Annual Performance Review Report 2020–21*. Nairobi, Kenya. Division of Health Sector Monitoring and Evaluation, MoH.

Kenya Ministry of Health (2023) *MoH Guidelines, Standards and Policies Portal*. http://guidelines. health.go.ke/#/ (accessed 09/2023).

Kenya Ministry of Health/WHO/World Bank (2013) *An Assessment of Patient Safety Standards in Kenya: Summary Report of Patient Safety survey*. https://uasingishureproductivehealth. files.wordpress.com/2015/08/kenya-patient-safety-survey-report-2014.pdf.

Khadiagala, G (2023) Kenya's political elites switch parties with every election – how this fuels violence. *The Conversation*. May 16, 2023. https://theconversation.com/.

Kimani, N (2020) *Meeting the Promise of the 2010 Constitution: Devolution, Gender and Equality in Kenya*. London. Chatham House. The Royal Institute of International Affairs.

Koumamba, A, Bisvigou, U, Ngoungou, E and Diallo, D (2021) Health information systems in developing countries: case of African countries, *BMC Medical Informatics and Decision-Making*, vol. 21, no. 1, 232–242.

Krah, E, de Kruijf, J and Ragno, L (2018) Integrating traditional healers into the health care system: challenges and opportunities in rural Northern Ghana, *Journal of Community Health*, vol. 43, 157–163.

Krüger, C, Heinzel-Gutenbrunner, M and Ali, M (2017) Adherence to the IMCI guidelines in Namibia, Kenya, Tanzania and Uganda: evidence from the national service provision assessment surveys, *BMC Health Services Research*, vol. 17, article number 822.

Kumah, E et al (2021) Framework for assessing the performance of the Ghanaian health system, *Health Research Policy and Systems*, vol. 19, 149.

Leo, C (1981) Who benefited from the million-Acre scheme? Toward a class analysis of Kenya's transition to independence, *Canadian Journal of African Studies/Revue*, vol. 15, no. 2, 201–222.

Martin, J (2022) *The Meddlers: Sovereignty, Empire, and the Birth of Global Economic Governance*. Cambridge, MA. Harvard University Press.

Mathauer, I, Saksena, P and Kutzin, J (2019) Pooling arrangements in health financing systems: a proposed classification, *International Journal for Equity in Health*, vol. 18, 198.

Mbau, R et al (2023) Analysing the efficiency of health systems: a systematic review of the literature, *Applied Health Economics and Health Policy*, vol. 21, 205–224.

Mburu, F (1981) Socio-political imperatives in the history of health development in Kenya, *Social Science and Medicine*, vol. 15a, 521–527.

McGivern, G, Seruwagi, S, Wafula, P, Kiefer, T and Nakidde, C et al (2021) *Strengthening Health Professional Regulation in Kenya and Uganda: Research Findings Policy Brief*. Coventry. University of Warwick Business School Publications.

Medical and Dental Council of Ghana (2023) *Resources*. https://mdcghana.org (accessed 10/ 2023).

MOMENTUM (2023) *Integrated Management of Childhood Illness in Three Districts in Ghana: Successes, Challenges, and Opportunities.* Washington, DC. USAID MOMENTUM.

Mullei, K, Wafula, F and Goodman, C (2008) *Implementing IMCI in Kenya: Challenges and Recommendations.* Consortium for Research on Equitable Health Systems (CREHS). https://crehs.lshtm.ac.uk/downloads/publications.

Mwubu, G (1995) Health care reform in Kenya: a review of the process, *Health Policy*, vol. 32, 245–255.

Nabunnya, L (2022) *District Health Information Software 2 (DHIS2) and Immunisation: Country Case Study – Ghana.* healthenabled.org.

NHIA – National Health Insurance Authority of Ghana (2023) *National Health Insurance Scheme.* https://www.nhis.gov.gh (accessed 05/2023).

Ndege, P (2009) *Colonialism and its Legacies in Kenya.* Fulbright–Hays Group Project Abroad Lecture Program. http://africanphilanthropy.issuelab.org/resources/19699/19699.pdf (accessed 09/2023).

Nimako, B, Baiden, F and Awoonor-Williams, J (2020) Towards effective participation of the private health sector in Ghana's COVID-19 response, *Pan African Medical Journal*, vol. 35, Suppl 2, 47.

Nyangena, J et al (2021) Maturity assessment of Kenya's health information system interoperability readiness, *BMJ Health and Care Informatics*, vol. 28, no. 1, 1–7.

Nyawira, L et al (2023) Examining the influence of health sector coordination on the efficiency of county health systems in Kenya, *BMC Health Services Research*, vol. 23, 355.

OAU – Organisation of African Unity (2001) *Abuja Declaration on HIV/Aids, Tuberculosis, and other related infectious diseases.* https://au.int/sites/default/files/pages/32894-file-2001-abuja-declaration.pdf (accessed 09/2023).

Odei-Lartey, E, Prah, R and Anane, E et al (2020) Utilization of the national cluster of district health information system for health service decision-making in selected districts of the Brong Ahafo region in Ghana, *BMC Health Services Research*, vol. 20, 514. https://doi.org/10.1186/s12913-020-05349-5.

Omran, A (1971) The epidemiologic transition: a theory of the epidemiology of population change, *Milbank Memorial Fund Quarterly*, vol. 49, 509–538.

OPHI – Oxford Poverty and Human Development Initiative (2023) *Global MPI Country Briefing, June 2023: Ghana.* https://ophi.org.uk/wp-content/uploads/CB_GHA_2023.pdf.

Oraro-Lawrence, T and Wyss, K (2020) Policy levers and priority-setting in universal health coverage: a qualitative analysis of healthcare financing agenda setting in Kenya, *BMC Health Services Research*, vol. 20, 182.

Owusu Sarkode, A (2021) Effect of the National Health Insurance Scheme on healthcare utilization and out-of-pocket payment: evidence from GLSS 7, *Humanities and Social Science Communications*, vol. 8, no. 293, 1–10.

Papanicolas, I, Rajan, D, Karanikolos, M and Figueras, J (2022) 'Assessing health systems performance for universal health coverage: rationale and approach' in Papanicolas, I, Rajan, D, Karanikolos, M, Soucat, A and Figueras, J (eds) *Health System Performance Assessment: A Framework for Policy Analysis.* European Observatory on Health Systems and Policy/WHO, pp 1–7.

Republic of Ghana Ministry of Finance (2021) *Press Release.* April 14. https://mofep.gov.gh/press-release/2021-04-14/ghana-has-not-been-down-graded-as-a-low-income-country (accessed 06/2023).

Rodríguez, D et al (2023) Political economy analysis of subnational health management in Kenya, Malawi and Uganda, *Health Policy and Planning*, vol. 38, 631–647.

Rondinelli, D (1981) Government decentralization in comparative perspective: theory and practice in developing countries, *International Review of Administrative Sciences*, vol. 47, 364–372.

Rose, G (1981) Strategy of prevention: lessons from cardiovascular disease, *British Medical Journal*, no. 282, 1847–1851.

Sumah, A, Bowan, P and Insah, B (2014) Decentralization in the Ghana health service: a study of the Upper West Region, *Developing Country Studies*, vol. 4, no. 12, 45–52.

Titi-Ofei, R, Osei-Afriyie, D and Karamagi, H (2021) Monitoring quality of care in the WHO Africa Region: a study design for measurement and tracking, *Global Health Action*, vol. 14, no. 1, 1939493.

Top, M, Konca, M and Sapaz, B (2020) Technical efficiency of healthcare systems in African countries: an application based on data envelopment analysis, *Health Policy and Technology*, vol. 9, no. 1, 62–68.

UNICEF (2023) *Countdown to 2030: Women's, Children, and Adolescents Health 2023.* https://data.unicef.org/countdown-2030 (accessed 01/2024).

United Nations (1997) *Agenda for Development – General Assembly – Resolution 51/240.* https://www.un.org (accessed 02/2023).

United Nations (2015) *Transforming our World: The 2030 Agenda for Sustainable Development.* https://www.un.org (accessed 06/2023).

United Nations (2021) *LDC's at a Glance.* Department of Economic and Social Affairs. https://www.un.org (accessed 04/2023).

United Nations (2022) *World Economic Situation and Prospects – Statistical Index.* https://www.un.org (accessed 04/2023).

United Nations Development Programme (2023a) *Explore the Human Development Index.* https://hdr.undp.org/data-center/human-development-index#/indicies/HDI (accessed 07/2023).

United Nations Development Programme (2023b) *Global Multi-dimensional Poverty Index 2023: Unstacking Global Poverty.* UNDP and Oxford Poverty and Human Development Initiative. https://hdr.undp.org (accessed 01/2024).

Wamai, R (2009) 'Healthcare policy and administration and reforms in post-colonial Kenya and challenges for the future' in Veintie, T and Virtanen, P (eds) *Local and Global Encounters: Norms, Identities and Representations in Formation.* Helsinki. Renvall Institute Publications 25.

Wang, H, Otoo, N and Dsane-Selby, L (2017) *Ghana National Health Insurance Scheme: Improving Financial Sustainability Based on Expenditure Review: A World Bank Study.* Washington, DC. World Bank Group.

World Bank (2022) *World Development Indicators Database.* Washington, DC. http://data.worldbank.org (accessed 05/2023).

World Bank (2023a) *The World Bank in Gabon.* Report. March 24, 2023. https://data.worldbank.org (accessed 05/2023).

World Bank (2023b) *The World Bank in Ghana.* Report. March 31, 2023. https://data.worldbank.org (accessed 05/2023).

World Bank (2023c) *The World Bank in Kenya.* Report. September 19, 2023. https://data.worldbank.org (accessed 10/2023).

World Health Organisation (1978) *Primary Health Care: Report of the International Conference on Primary Health Care, Alma-Ata, USSR, 6–12 September 1978.* https://www.who.int/publications/i/item/9241800011.

World Health Organisation (1995) *World Health Organization Traditional Practitioners as Primary Health Care Workers: A Study of Effectiveness of Four Training Projects in Ghana, Mexico and Bangladesh.* Geneva. WHO.

World Health Organisation (2005) *International Health Regulations* (3rd Ed). Geneva, Switzerland. WHO.

World Health Organisation (2013) *WHO Traditional Medicine Strategy 2014–2023.* Geneva. WHO.

World Health Organisation (2015) *Service Availability and Readiness Assessment (SARA): Implementation Guide and Reference Manual – Version 2:2.* Geneva. WHO.

World Health Organisation (2017) *Half the World lacks access to essential health services.* Press Release. December 13, 2017. www.who.int.

World Health Organisation (2021a) *Global Patient Safety Action Plan 2021–2030: Towards Eliminating Avoidable Harm in Health Care.* Geneva. Switzerland. WHO.

World Health Organisation (2021b) *IHR 2005 – States Parties Self-Assessment Annual Reporting Tool* (2nd Ed). Geneva, Switzerland. WHO.

World Health Organisation (2022) *Global Expenditure on Health: Rising to the Pandemics Challenges.* Geneva, Switzerland. WHO.

World Health Organisation (2023a) *Global Health Observatory – indicators.* https://who.int/data/gho (accessed 09/2023).

World Health Organisation (2023b) *Health Topics – International Health Regulations.* https://www.who.int (accessed 12/2023).

World Health Organisation (2024a) *The Global Health Observatory – IHR (2005) SPAR Second Edition – Country Data Tables*. https://www.who.int (accessed 06/2024).

World Health Organisation (2024b) *Child Health and Development Unit – Integrated management of childhood illness*. https://www.who.int (accessed 06/2024).

World Health Organisation Ghana (2022) *Annual Report*. Accra, Ghana. WHO.

World Health Organisation, Regional Office for Africa (2022) *Atlas of African Health Statistics*. https://aho.afro.who.int/publications (accessed 08/2023).

World Health Organisation, Regional Office for Africa (2023a) *National Health Observatories*. https://aho.afro.who.int/data-by-country/af (accessed 08/2023).

World Health Organisation, Regional Office for Africa (2023b) *Health Topics/Immunization*. https://www.afro.who.int/health-topics/immunization (accessed 01/2024).

World Health Organisation, Regional Office for Africa (2023c) *Technical Efficiency of Health Systems in the WHO African Region*. WHO African Region Brazzaville, Congo. WHO Regional Office for Africa.

World Health Organisation, Regional Office for Europe (2022) *European Health for All Database*. https://gateway.euro.who.int/en/datasets/european-health-for-all-database/ (accessed 02/2023).

Young, C (2004) The end of the post-colonial state in Africa? Reflections on changing African political dynamics, *African Affairs*, vol. 103, 23–49.

CHAPTER 7

Germany and the UK

A comparative analysis of health systems in high-income countries

Historical background to the development of the NHS in Britain

The National Health Service (NHS) founded in 1948, replaced a disorganised pre-war mixture of charitable, local government, and private market provision with a national system that provided universal health care coverage for the first time to the population. In the early decades following the end of the war a political consensus existed which was predicated on the understanding that the most effective and the fairest means of ensuring that health care was available for all was through a state-organised system funded from direct taxation. But how and why did this radical departure from what had existed before come about?

Answering this question requires a historical overview that begins in the mid-nineteenth century, with the establishment of the decentralised system of 'Poor Law' relief for the poor and the destitute. These reforms were predicated on the doctrine of 'less eligibility' promoted by the social reformer, Edwin Chadwick, this ensured that any relief (or subsidies) that were provided by local parishes must be worked for by its recipients. This was a significant departure from the charitable principles of alms-giving, reflecting the social and economic changes that were then occurring in the newly industrialised areas of Britain. Local parishes (prior to the establishment of modern forms of local government) were encouraged to establish factory-like 'workhouses', where poor families as well as the sick were housed. Those who were able were required to work for their 'relief' that was set at a level below the standard living of those in employment. Life in the workhouse, which was starkly portrayed in many of the novels of Charles Dickens, was characterised by appalling and desperate conditions for the families incarcerated there. Yet, the Poor Law system did establish local infirmaries and rudimentary hospitals for the 'sick poor', these institutions could be said to constitute the first publicly funded forms of health care provision. It was to take many decades more before there was any further significant intervention by the British state in the organisation of health care provision.

In 1919, following the ending of the First World War, a Ministry of Health was established for the first time. This new Department of State was charged with the task of integrating the disparate provision of health care in Britain, particularly in relation to child and maternity care. The health care provision that did exist at the time was organised by range of often localised organisations, some were charities, some were 'voluntary'/philanthropic, the long-established parish Poor Law infirmaries were still

DOI: 10.4324/9781003564249-10

in existence, and there were the private hospitals that were open only to fee-paying patients. Primary care was essentially non-existent. There were doctors who practised in the community, but these worked as private traders (noting that General Practice as a medical speciality was not established until the founding of the NHS in 1948). There were also an array of community-based nurses and midwives; these were also employed by a range of institutions including religious charities, Metropolitan Boards of Health, as well as the parishes administering the Poor Law system. In combination, this provision did not constitute an organised and effective system of community nursing. In 1929, local borough councils were empowered to take over all the existing Poor Law infirmaries, but few of these authorities, outside of London, were in a financial position to develop new 'municipal' hospitals. Between 1921 and 1938, the public provision of hospital beds increased by only 4,000 reaching a total of just 176,000 beds. The 'Voluntary' hospital sector that was composed primarily of the main teaching hospitals, with independent status thanks to philanthropic and other private sources of funding, provided a further 87,000 beds (Fraser:1973;186). The Ministry of Health struggled to make any impression at all in bringing about any semblance of integration of this disparate range of provision during this interwar period.

A political consensus for more radical reform of health care provision began to emerge during the 1930s in the face of economic depression and rising unemployment. But it was the outbreak of the Second World War in 1939 that finally gave this process a dramatic push forward. At the very beginning of hostilities, the government set-up the Emergency Hospital Service (EHS) to coordinate the work of all hospitals, private and local government in anticipation of mass civilian bombing casualties that would result from the mass bombing of cities. By 1941, the Ministry of Health announced that it had commissioned the economist William Beveridge to produce a report examining the ways in which a comprehensive social security and health care system could be created after the war. The Beveridge Report was published in 1942, and, it proposed the creation of a national 'welfare state' that would provide a minimum standard of living 'below which no one should be allowed to fall' and a 'National Health Service' providing medical treatment for 'all citizens'.[1]

A key recommendation of the Beveridge Report was the application of the principle of universalism to be applied to the proposed new state pension and unemployment benefit, as well as to the provision of health care services. Nevertheless, some pre-war attitudes did persist, and means-testing of the incomes of families would continue to determine their access to additional social protection benefits up to and including the present day. The application of the principle of universalism was to be tempered by economic reality; 'affordability' (for the system) rather than 'need' (of the population) became a defining institutional feature of health and welfare provision. Unusually for an official government report, the Ministry of Information made the decision to give extensive media publicity to the Beveridge Report and its recommendations. The report was widely distributed and sold over a hundred thousand copies, an unprecedented event in British policy-making. The Report was also circulated to the armed forces in the field, 'as a means of showing what those fighting for the country might return to' (Greener & Powell:2021;277).

Thelan (1999) identifies the historic role of what he terms 'change-agents' in government policy-making; these are people and organisations able to counter the preexisting status quo ('vetoing tendencies') of state systems. William Beveridge can be seen as a pre-eminent 'change agent'. His report was in tune with a popular demand for radical reform during the uncertainty and collective hardship of war, and challenged many of the pre-war vested interests involved in health care provision. These included the medical consultants and General Practitioners (GPs) many of whom had lucrative private health practices, the PHI companies, as well as the Voluntary hospital sector, all of which had long blocked any reform to the pre-war health care system. But following the Labour Party's landslide victory in the post-war general election of 1945, a government was now elected that had a democratic mandate to construct a to new form of welfare state on the lines broadly proposed by Beveridge.

The post-war NHS in Britain

The NHS came into full operation in July 1948, following the National Health Service Act of 1946. The new organisation effectively nationalised some 1,143 voluntary hospitals with 90,000 beds, and 1,545 local municipally run hospitals with 390,000 beds, of which 190,000 were in mental illness and 'mental deficiency' (which we would now term 'intellectual disability') asylums. The funding of the NHS was to come through general taxation. Here it should be noted that the system of National Insurance contributions that was established at the same time has only ever representing a fraction of the total cost of operating all the state institutions of welfare, including the NHS. The organisational structure of the new NHS was a 'tripartite' one, and in part this reflected the compromises and concessions made to the medical profession (discussed below). National health care provision was now to be divided between primary (preventative, involving GPs), secondary (acute medicine, located in the Hospital sector), and tertiary (care of chronically ill).

During the final stages of the legislation process, important concessions were granted to the medical establishment to ensure their participation in the new system. Doctors in General Practice (the new GP training programme was being instigated at this time) were able to retain their privileged position as independent contractors and were not to become state employees, while hospital consultants were also able to continue their lucrative private practice, working only for a minimal amount of hours per week within the new NHS. Far from challenging the position of authority that the medical profession had enjoyed in the pre-war system, new powers were now ceded to them, particularly in relation to the health resource allocation process. These compromises established a self-regulated autonomy for the profession that it was to retain for decades. The decision-making control over health spending that was ceded to senior members of the medical profession inevitably led to an inequitable distribution of resources across the NHS. The profession ensured that the lion's share of resources went to the elite teaching hospitals, mainly located in London (where there were 12), Edinburgh, and Manchester. Outside of the main teaching hospitals as was argued at the time, twentieth-century medicine was being practised in nineteenth-century buildings, a legacy of the underfunded, ill-equipped, and unevenly distributed pre-war provision of health services.

The average annual increase in health care spending in Britain in the period 1948–60 was just 2%, although this increased to 5% a year from the mid-1960s onwards (Health Foundation:2015). It was only from this period on that the UK economy was finally in a sufficiently financially stable position, following the requirements of post-war debt maintenance and infrastructural re-organisation, to enable the government to find the additional funds necessary to embark on an extensive hospital building programme to address regional inequities. The 1962 Hospital Plan set out guidelines for the development of new and larger 'District Hospitals', as well introducing new layers of specialist managers and greater specialisation of hospital support services. A new commitment to rationalising the organisation of NHS services was reflected in the introduction of strategic planning for the primary care services. Yet nearly 20 years after the founding of the NHS, some 33 million people were still considered to be living in what were described as 'undoctored' areas, notably in inner city and rural areas (Ham:1992;20).

On this basis of this belated recognition of unmet health care needs, the Labour government established the Merrison Commission in 1976 to look into ways of improving efficiency in the management of NHS financial and human resources. The Commission's Report was published in 1979 and identified a widening of the social and geographical inequalities in health across the UK, while also recognising that this was a social problem that could not be addressed by the health care system in isolation from other branches of government (Merrison:1979). In 1979, the incoming Conservative government chose to largely ignore the recommendations of the Merrison Report.[2]

Reforming the NHS: 1979–2008

The election of the Conservative government headed by Margaret Thatcher, an early adopter of neoliberal[3] economic thinking, represented an ideological challenge to the post-war consensus that held to the necessity of a universal state-financed health care. Initially, the new government held back from enacting any extensive structural reforms to the NHS, while at the same time engaging in significant privatising reforms to other sectors of the welfare state, including social security, education, and housing. This reluctance to intervene in the NHS reflected the high levels of popular support it enjoyed from the public, re-organising the health system it was feared would damage the government's political credibility. But finally, nearly a decade since first being elected Prime Minister, Margaret Thatcher announced, via an interview broadcast on the BBC *Panorama* current affairs programme in January 1988, that she was setting-up a high-level review into the organisational structuring of the NHS. The outcome of this review when it was completed was the *Working for Patients* White Paper published in January 1989.

The proposals for organisational change that were set out in the White Paper were described by the Prime Minister herself at the time, 'as the most far-reaching reform of the NHS in its forty year history' (Webster:2002;190). What subsequently became known as 'the internal market' reforms were intended to promote the introduction of market forces within the organisation of the NHS. The underpinning neo-liberal rationale was that promoting competition by separating the purchasing of health care services from its provision, would improve efficiency and reduce costs. GP's practices were now to become 'fund-holders' and to use the monies allocated to them by central government to them to purchase health services on behalf of their patients within newly created hospital 'Trusts'. The latter were to compete with one another to provide health care services, with payments 'following the patient'. The reaction to the publication of the White Paper from the health care professions was one of generalised and vociferous condemnation, described at the time, as the 'biggest explosion of political anger and professional fury in the history of the NHS' (Klein:1995;131). The British Medical Association (BMA) launched a campaign of opposition (much had changed in the profession over the forty years since it had opposed the introduction of the NHS) supported by the other health service trade unions, as well as the Labour Party. Nevertheless, no concessions were forthcoming from the government, and the *NHS & Community Care Act* that embodied the reforms was passed into law in 1990.

The unsupported claim made by the government that these reforms to the organisation of the NHS would facilitate 'patient power' proved to be a largely spurious one (Paton:2014;5). It was not so much a question of the patient dictating where funding went, and more one of the patient 'following whatever channel the professionals dictated' (Webster:2002;202). This organisational reform occurred at a time when the UK had been out of official economic recession for nearly a decade[4] (ONS:2015), reinforcing the point that these reforms were driven more by ideology than fiscal necessity. Yet even as the 'internal market' reforms were being implemented, doubts began to rise about the extent of the government's commitment to rigorously pursue their ideological goals. As Rudolf Klein has noted: '(T)he notion driving these changes was that competition among providers to secure contracts either from the Health Authorities or from general practitioners who chose to be fund-holders would improve efficiency and responsiveness. For a variety of reasons, among them the reluctance of the government to give free rein to market forces, the reforms never functioned as intended' (Klein:2001;937).

If a privatised NHS did not emerge from these reforms, then a new organisational structure certainly did. One of its enduring legacies was the introduction of what became known as the 'New Public Management' (NPM).[5] The NPM was described at the time as constituting, 'the injection of an ideological "foreign body" into a sector previously characterized by quite different traditions of thought' (Pollitt:1995;136). The traditional division of labour within the NHS, long marked by hierarchal lines of authority, was now to be transformed, and the new model of management and work relations began to 'mirror capitalist organization and techniques' (Carter:2020;148). When the 'New' Labour government finally returned to government under the premiership of Tony Blair in 1997, it did not end the separation of health service purchasing from provision. Rather, it set about establishing its own slimmed down version of market-based reforms, this it termed 'modernisation'. But as Bob Carter has also noted, this was 'a deliberately disarming concept, suggesting technicality and value-neutrality' (Carter:2020;149).

The New Labour government set out its own programme for NHS reform in its White Paper, *The New NHS: Modern, dependable* (DoH:1997). The stated objective of this programme was to move away from promoting outright market 'competition' but rather to promote the benefits of market 'incentives' in order to improve efficiency of the service. This phrasing masked what was essentially a semantic divergence only from the previous government's market-influenced reforms. Health care financing was no longer to 'follow the patient', but the provider-purchaser separation was maintained. A system of 'commissioning' by newly created Primary Care Groups (PCGs) was established, replacing the GP fundholding system. A further objective for these PCGs, later to be termed Primary Care Trusts (PCTs), was to take on a greater range of strategic community health planning. Although the PCGs were formally multi-disciplinary bodies, they remained largely dominated by GPs (Paton:2006). Subsequent developments saw the expansion of 'Foundation Hospital Trusts', these were acute general hospitals and mental health trusts which were now required to 'pass' a series of performance tests of financial and organisational competence in order to gain their new status. As such they were able to formally operate as independent, but publicly financed, providers of secondary health care. Finally, the private health care sector was enabled, through the new commissioning process, to formally compete to be providers of secondary, primary, and long-term care services.

The primary focus of the New Labour government reforms, or so it was claimed, was to achieving 'an efficient and equitable' health service. New efficiency standards were introduced within the organisational structures of the NHS, and these were monitored and regulated through the introduction of new dedicated digital health information and management systems. Roles were also created for two new 'arms-length bodies'.[6] One was the Commission for Health improvement, which subsequently became known as the Health Care Commission from 2004–08, and is today known as the Care Quality Commission (CQA). This body was charged with carrying out regular monitoring and inspection of all health care providers to ensure that clinical standards were being met and maintained. The second ALB was the National Institute of Clinical Excellence (NICE), known since 2013 as the National Institute for Health and Care Excellence,[7] but it has retained the same acronym. This body carries out what are known as 'technology appraisals' of new pharmaceuticals, diagnostic equipment, and other medical technologies. It has also established over the course of two decades, national guidance for clinical interventions for a broad range of medical conditions (known as the 'Quality Outcomes Framework').

Although health system 'efficiency' remained defined primarily in 'value-for-money' terms, one of the key points of divergence from the approach of the previous Conservative regime was that the New Labour government did succeed in constructing an effective regulatory system of governance[8] for clinical professional practice as well as for patient safety. This enhanced oversight capacity was in theory reinforced by clear lines of managerial control over the day-to-day running of the health service. However, as patient safety and care scandals began to emerge over the following decade, it was clear that the system of governance went only so far. For example, there were never any accountability structures put in place to ensure that the regulators themselves were regulated.

A House of Commons Select Committee Report (HoC:2010) published the year that New Labour were voted out of office, noted that this new organisational network has resulted in an increase in the administrative costs (reoccurring annual costs) of the NHS in England from 5% of its total budget in the late 1980s to 14% in 2005. It is important to note that the NHS had previously always been held up as an exemplary example of sustaining low administrative cost in comparison to health care systems with private market and social insurance funding mechanisms (Paton:2014;7). The increase in administrative costs aside, over the course of the decade 1997 to 2007 (the year the global banking and financial markets crash upended state fiscal spending), public spending on health care increased from 5% to 8% of GDP (see the data presented in Figure 7.1), equating to an average 6.3% yearly increase in real terms (Lloyd:2015). This positively reflected the New Labour Party's electoral commitment in 1997 to increase health spending so that it was comparable with the Western European average. It should also be noted that economic growth across in the UK in this period averaged over 3.5% per annum (World Bank:2022), which certainly provided favourable conditions for achieving this objective.

Finally it should be noted that the New Labour government also acceded to its electoral commitment to the creation of devolved authorities in Scotland, Northern Ireland and Wales. This process involved the transfer of a range of powers, including responsibility for health care provision, from Westminster, the seat of the UK government, to the Scottish Parliament, Welsh Senedd, and the Northern Ireland assembly in Stormont in 1999. These devolved administrations now received a 'block grant' for public spending from the UK government, and were given the organisational autonomy to determine health spending priorities within the overarching framework of NHS universal provision. The existence of separate health administrations in each of the four nations constituting the UK did predate the 1999 devolution reforms, going back to the foundation of the NHS in 1948. However, the difference was that previously, centralised UK government departments directly managed what were conceived as being regional areas in a national system.

Austerity and yet more reform: the NHS from 2008 to the present day

On coming into office in 2010, the Coalition government (Conservative and Liberal Democrat) chose to embrace and expand the fiscal austerity politics that the New Labour government had resorted to following the 2008 global banking crises and the economic recession that followed. This was despite the fact that by 2010, the world economy was slowly beginning a period of recovery. Under these circumstances, the textbook macroeconomic approach would be to embark upon a programme of fiscal stimulus, yet the Coalition government eschewed this orthodoxy and chose to do the opposite, reducing the scale of state fiscal support for the UK economy. This continuation of austerity was to have long-term consequences for the NHS. Serial underinvestment in the health service (as well as other key arms of the welfare state) has ultimately served to undermine the universality of health care provision in Britain as NHS waiting times for treatment were to increase threefold over the course of the following 14 years of Conservative government stewardship.

Alongside the austerity politics, the Conservative-led government returned to their ideological project of opening-up the NHS to market forces, setting about the construction of what would be in effect the third round of health system organisational reforms since 1990. The passing of the *Health and Social Care Act* in 2012 represented a legislative shift from what had been the previous statutory obligation, 'to *provide* or secure a comprehensive health service', which was now to be reduced to, 'a duty to *promote* a comprehensive health service' (Health and Social Care Act:2012); an important distinction in Law. This legislative change in effect removed the statutory responsibility for the health care of citizens from the Minister of State for Health, a role that the responsible minister had held continually since the founding of the NHS in 1948. While the formal responsibility for budgeting, planning, delivery, and the day-to-day operation of health services was passed onto a newly created non-departmental ALB, the NHS Commissioning Board Authority, which was renamed 'NHS England' the following year, 2013.

The 2012 legislation also strengthened the system of local commissioning, this followed the creation of Clinical Commissioning Groups (CCGs) which were headed up by GPs, replacing the previous multi-disciplinary PCT's. Simultaneously all health care providers (for-profit, voluntary or NHS), were placed in direct competition against each other, through the introduction of what became known as the 'Any Qualified Provider' mechanism, an example of the process of marketisation at work within the NHS. The reforms to the commissioning system also resulted in a significant splintering of local NHS institutions, despite the fact that prior to the reforms it was known that the evident gaps in health care equity and service delivery were directly due to the lack of collaboration and cohesiveness between local health care organisations. By making the local CCGs health care purchasers as well as giving them the responsibility for providing a population-level public health system, the 2012 organisational reforms created the potential to further attribute any shortfall in primary care provision 'to bad local management rather than bad central government' (Speed & Gabe:2020;35).

This drive to impose further organisational reform was driven as much by the fiscal politics of 'austerity' as it was by the continuing influence of a neoliberal ideology committed to state retrenchment. This was a further attempt to impose a Hayekian[9] model of 'small government' acting as a neutral commissioner or 'broker' of health and welfare services in a free market of providers, alongside a decentralised residual system of service provision for the 'deserving poor'. The impact of this political strategy on health spending was a flattening of any real term increase. By 2014, it was estimated by NHS England itself, that the cost of meeting the predictable increase in health care needs over the period 2013/14 to 2020/21 would cost £30bn more than the government was willing to commit itself to over the next decade (NHS England:2014). The failure to achieve any real term increase in government health spending by 2021, in comparison with the previous two decades, is clearly apparent in Figure 7.1.

The COVID-19 pandemic struck in early 2020. The government responded with a temporary and ring-fenced increase in health spending that accounted for approximately £50bn additional spending in both 2020–21 and in 2021–22 (but note that in order to represent the historical trend in UK health spending, the additional COVID-19 funding is not included in the data for 2021/22 set out in Figure 7.1). The additional COVID-19 spending ceased in the financial year 2022/23. In the midst of the pandemic, at a time when the NHS was stretched beyond its capacity to treat patients safety, the Conservative government under Boris Johnson's premiership, and now in its 12th year of power, introduced legislation for Parliamentary approval that proposed yet still further structural reforms to the provision and delivery of health care in the England, the fourth round of major reforms undertaken since 1990. In April 2022, the *Health and Care Act* received Royal Assent, with the main thrust of this legislation designed to provide a formal framework to support what the government termed 'collaboration and partnership-working', with the goal of improving the integration of primary care services for patients. These 'Integrated Care Services' (ICSs) are at the centre of these most recent structural reforms to the NHS (see Figure 7.2).

ICSs are intended to constitute a new regional structural layer, with each one serving on average some 2 million people. They have effectively replaced the GP-led CCGs as budget-holders, tasked with planning and commissioning local-regional health services. The legislation requires the regional ICSs meet four key objectives: (a) improve population health and health care outcomes, (b) address in health outcomes, experience, and access, (c) improve productivity and value for money, (d) contribute to supporting broader regional social and economic development. Two newly created

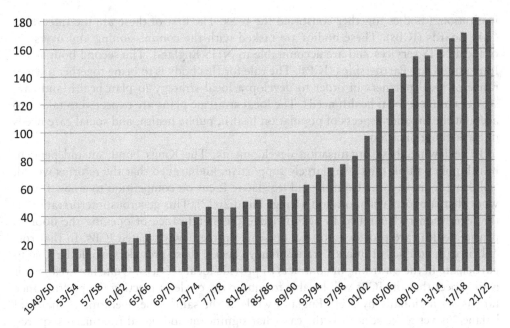

Figure 7.1 HM treasury public expenditure on health 1949–2021 real terms spending £bn 2022/23 prices (Adapted from BMA (2023)).

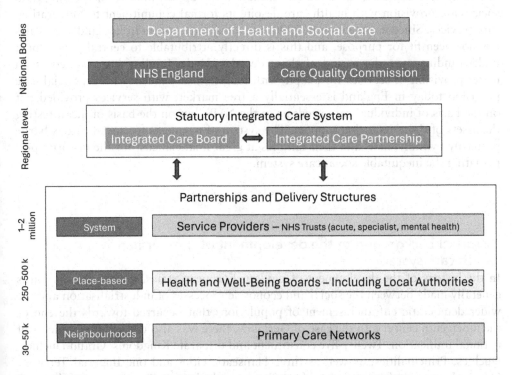

Figure 7.2 The structure of the NHS in England (Health and Care Act (2022)).

institutional bodies together constitute the ICSs. The first of these are the Integrated Care Boards (ICBs). These bodies are tasked with the commissioning and oversight of local NHS services and are accountable to NHS England. The second body is the Integrated Care Partnerships (ICPs). The role for this body is to bring together a wider range of local partners in order to develop a local strategy to plan health and care services to meet local health needs. The local strategic plans are expected to take into account the broader aspects of population health, public health, and social care needs of the local population.

In reviewing these organisation developments, The Kings Fund, an independent health policy think tank, was largely supportive, and argued that the reforms would, 'solidify the move away from the old legislative focus on competition to a new framework that supports collaboration' (Kings Fund:2022). This generous interpretation of the legislation rather failed to acknowledge the significance of opening the door to private health care providers to take up seats on the newly created ICBs. In that role (albeit with conflict of interest transparency checks) these providers would be able to participate in the awarding of contracts to provide local services. Quite how realistic it is to expect that the ICBs will be able to square the circle of meeting the performance targets set nationally by NHS England while at the same time operating a 'financial balance' is yet to be seen. It is the case that significant additional funding is required if ICBs are able to meet the challenge of establishing 'integrated' partnerships between local authorities and local voluntary and community enterprise sectors, with the goal of developing regional strategies to tackle inequalities, improve local health outcomes, and support social and economic development.

Finally and not least, the 2022 Act eschewed the opportunity to merge long-term social care provision with health care despite its formal commitment to 'integrating' care services. Since its inception in 1990, the social care system in England and Wales has not been fit for purpose, and this is directly attributable to central government under-funding over the period of three decades. Under-funding has resulted in an under-provision of services for people with long-term dependency needs. Social care provision today in England is essentially a free market, with services provided not on the basis of individual care needs as in the NHS, but on the basis of mean-testing the assets of those requiring support. The system of payments for social care is borne primarily by individuals and their families at great financial cost for the majority perpetuating the inequitable social care system.

****

Historical background to the development of the German health care system

In the history of the development of modern European states, a close association is generally made between the social and economic processes of industrialisation and the wider democratic enfranchisement of populations that occurred towards the end of the nineteenth century. In the case of Germany, there was also the additional factor of national unification. Twenty-five constituent and disparate Kingdoms, Grand Duchies, Duchies, Principalities, as well as three Hanseatic cities and one Imperial Territory (Alsace-Lorraine), the latter seized from France in the Franco-Prussian war of the same year, came together under one national state in 1871. The newly unified German state, under the leadership of the Chancellor, Otto Von Bismarck, was immediately pressurised by both employer's associations, as well as the organised labour movement demanding, 'positive measures to deal with the pathological features of industrial society' (Rosenhaft:1994;30).

A growing class of industrial workers were now migrating in large numbers from the rural areas of the country to the new factories in the expanding industrial cities of Germany. What concerned both employers and workers was that traditional forms of community and charitable support, especially in the case of sickness and frailty, were being lost in the twin processes of industrialisation and urbanisation. Both groups urged the new German State to establish systems of social protection to compensate for this loss. In 1883, the state responded to these demands when it introduced its ground-breaking (in European not just German terms) health and social insurance legislation in 1883. This compulsorily mandated both employees and employers to make regular contributions to cover sickness and industrial injury. These contributions were to be paid into the pre-existing local voluntary medical and social health insurance (SHI) funding schemes, now subject to regulation by the national state. In the geographical areas where these schemes did not previously exist, the law now required the creation of new schemes. Mandatory insurance to cover invalidity and old age pensions was not introduced until 1889, with a direct funding role played by the state. The 1883 legislation is often seen as constituting the basis of a future German welfare state, but in practice it represented only a minimal interventionary role for the new state, limited to the provision of a framework of legal compulsion, and administrative terms of reference for the pre-existing SHI schemes (Rosenhaft:1994;31). The social protection interventions should not be seen as the act of a beneficent state and an enlightened political establishment. Bismarck himself stated that his reforms were introduced as an explicit political bribe to shift the allegiances of an increasingly radicalised and organised working class away from the influence of socialist political parties and trade unions, and aimed at 'tying workers to the state by providing welfare benefits' (Zöllner:1982;13 – cited in Moran:1999;45). In this respect Bismarck was ultimately unsuccessful in that the popular vote for the Social Democratic Party that represented the organised working class continued to rise, and by 1912 it was the largest party in the German Parliament, the Reichstag.

However, the bureaucratic organisation of this expanding health and welfare insurance system did establish the right of workers to have direct representation in the administration of local SHI funds (Rosenhaft:1994;32). Prior to the 1883 legislation, local SHI schemes paid-out benefits in cash directly to their members, which could then be used as income maintenance whilst sick or spent on any variety of health provision, not necessarily doctors. Whereas, in the post-1883 statutory insurance system, these local funding schemes were now required to pay doctors directly for health services provided to members. This had the consequence of ensuring a significant new income for the medical profession which bound them directly to the SHI funds, and 'in this entanglement lies a key to the subsequent historical development of the whole system' (Moran:1999;35). This aspect of German public administration which served to limit the direct role of the central state and the market in health care provision was later to develop into a defining feature of the post-Second World War German welfare state that became widely known as 'corporatism'.

Health outcomes for the German working class undoubtedly improved following the introduction of statutory SHI schemes. However, the question that has been posed is whether this improvement reflected the widening access to health care combined with the security of sickness insurance, or more general improvements in the standard of living that were then occurring in Germany. Recent research by Bauernschuster et al (2020) draws on newly digitised administrative data from Prussia, the largest of the German states in the period following the introduction of the 1883 legislation. These authors were able to analyse the local district level annual occupation-specific mortality rates, for the period 1877–1900. Their conclusions were that SHI did indeed reduce blue-collar workers' mortality by 8.9% in this period, accounting for approximately a third of the overall mortality decline of industrial workers.

The Bismarckian SHI funding schemes continued to operate in broadly the same way after the First World War and into the 'Great Depression' of the late 1920s. By 1925, 51% of the German population were insured, represented by some 7,777 separate medical insurance sickness funds; health expenditure having tripled since 1884. Yet SHI-funded provision of health services remained fragmentary. Ambulatory or out-patient services (both terms are used interchangeably in the literature) were delivered by 'office-based' doctors, members of associations that held a monopoly over the distribution of regional sickness funds. This served to effectively separate ambulatory care from in-patient hospital care (Blümel et al:2020;17). The reforms enacted during the Weimar governments of the inter-war period served to strengthen still further the autonomy of the medical profession funded by the SHI schemes, weakening the administrative role played by the Trade Unions. During the Nazi Dictatorship in Germany, the founding principles of SHI funding were significantly distorted. The role of the funds as independent political actors was ended, and state-appointed officials appointed to administer them. The Nazis gave the medical profession control over the resources of the compulsory funds, 'reshaping the regulatory relationship between the profession and the state' (Moran:1999;37). Access to health care was now to be denied to Germany's Jewish population, and Jewish doctors, who constituted over 50% of the profession in Berlin in 1933, were prohibited from practising medicine. Millions of Jewish people were subsequently murdered in the Nazi death camps.

West German post-war reconstruction

By the end of the Second World War in 1945, the German economy and infrastructure was completely devastated. The country was now divided between the Western and Eastern power blocs following Germany's unconditional surrender. In addition, some 11 million ethnic German refugees and expellees, from nations such as Czechoslovakia, Hungary, and Romania, were now searching for security, homes, and jobs. The fast-track 'integration of these refugees and expellees into post war German society was surely one of the most remarkable features of the German recovery' (Evans:2024;180). Post-war reconstruction led directly to an enforced 'second round of capitalist transformation', a process which dismantled many of Germany's pre-war social, political, and economic structures, many of which pre-dated the Nazi regime, as they were seen to be holding back the progression of a modern capitalist economy (Anderson:2016). The newly formed *Bundesrepublik Deutschland* (BRD), also known in English as the Federal Republic of Germany (FRG), or more colloquially as West Germany, was a country much reduced in geographical size and population, and was in effective 'semi-sovereign' in domestic and international policy-making terms (Streek:2020;44). Indeed, up until 1949, West Germany was still divided into three occupied zones, controlled by the Americans, British, and the French. When this effective foreign occupation ended, the BRD adopted a new constitution (the 'Basic Law') that regulated central government intervention as well as giving significant authority and power (including health acre provision responsibilities) to the 16 federated *Länder* or regions.

The BRD was formally integrated into the post-war US-led 'Bretton-Woods' free trade agreement, this required member countries to guarantee convertibility of their currencies into US Dollars, which in turn gave that country much greater economic and fiscal security. These economic and financial developments 'laid the foundation for the re-establishment of a uniquely strong, heavily export-dependent industrial sector which was to become the centre of gravity of the West German and later the German political economy' (Streek:2020;46). This process became known as the *Wirtschaftswunder* or 'economic miracle', although there was nothing miraculous about the privation, sacrifices, and labour endured by the majority of German in the years following the ending of the war. By 1957, the BRD had became a core participant of the new European Economic Community (EEC), the forerunner to the European Union (EU).

Nevertheless, there was to be no fresh start, what was referred to as *Stunde null* or zero hour for the health and welfare system in the BRD, no dramatic reforms were made to the pre-war Bismarckian system. The opportunity to reform the system following the introduction of the 1949 'Basic Law' constitution was eschewed. The occupying Allied administration, and in particular the British, had in 1948 proposed a complete rationalisation of the system of health and social protection, following the principles set out in the Beveridge Plan. That is, the creation of a command-control type welfare state, providing universal benefits and health provision for all German citizens, regardless of income. But this Allied proposal was rejected in favour of continuity with the pre-war corporatist structures of social and health insurance, despite their known adequacies. Reforming the pre-war social insurance system was seen as a threat to the vested interests of private health and social insurance companies, as well as to the medical profession in their comfortable private practices. In addition, local artisan and agricultural organisations, industrialists, as well as middle level white-collar workers, also came together to block radical reform. Another explanation for the rejection of a centralised state health and welfare system points to an important difference in the German and British post-war experience: 'In Britain the war experience had engendered a sense of national solidarity and confidence in state intervention and had thus prepared the ground for the Beveridge reforms; in Germany, by contrast, the experience of Nazi misuse of power had provoked opposition to any form of government imposed centralisation or collectivism' (Hockerts:1981;318).

By the middle of the 1950s, 'an institutional structure had been rebuilt that strikingly resembled that created before 1939; indeed, it even included some features that were added in the Second World War' (Moran:1999;34). In 1952, the main opposition party in the German Parliament (*Bundestag*), the *Sozialdemokratische Partei* (SPD) or Social Democratic Party in English, did propose a motion to, 'appoint a kind of German Beveridge Committee, in order to prepare a comprehensive programme of social reform' (Hockerts:1981;323). However, the governing party, the *Christlich Demokratische Union* (CDU) or Christian Democrats in English, rejected the British blueprint and 'continued to stress the need for private initiative, for incentives and the individual's responsibility for his own security, and therefore sought to limit more narrowly the extent of government intervention' (Hockerts:1981;325). Any significant extension to the SHI system with its enshrined mechanisms of self-governance would have to wait until the reconstructed West German economy began to see dramatic growth from 1957 onwards.

The period between 1965 and 1975 saw significant improvements in the provision of health services, which continued to be funded through compulsory SHI schemes. In 1969, blue-collar industrial workers won the right to up to 6 weeks' full salary sick pay, although white-collar workers had enjoyed this sickness benefit since 1930! In 1970, preventive medical check-ups and paediatric screenings were included for the first time in the standard SHI benefits package. Further reforms in 1973 saw the introduction of the *Act to Improve Services* which removed the pre-existing time limited payments for hospital care as well as sick pay to compensate for wages lost while caring for a sick child. This legislation also extended the population coverage for rehabilitation services, as well as for dental and orthodontic services. As a consequence, SHI expenditure increased significantly over the course of this decade, measured as percentage of GDP, it went from 3.5% in 1965 to 5.9% in 1975. This was an outcome that was described at the time as the *Kostenexplosion im Gesundheitswesen* or 'cost explosion in health care' (Busse et al:2017;884).

Health costs were also to rise exponentially as a consequence of the global increase in prices that arose from the imposition of an oil embargo by the Organization of Arab Petroleum Exporting Countries (OAPEC) in 1973.[10] This 'crises' had a significant impact in slowing down the rates of economic growth, which in turn threatened the financial sustainability of SHI schemes. This effectively ended the on-going process of expanding health provision, and cuts in services and reductions in benefits soon followed. As a result, co-payments for health care services were introduced for the first time in 1977, these were payments additional to SHI contributions and were gradually extended into more and more areas of provision. The 1988 Health Care Reform Act increased co-payments for prescriptions, some forms of dental treatment, orthodontic treatment, transportation to and from medical facilities, and additional daily costs in-patient stays. As these indirect costs for health care increased, it became necessary to introduce exemption rules for people with high health expenditures related to long-term illness, and for those with limited household incomes. Increasing reliance on co-payments to fund health care ultimately meant that 'the economic consequences of illness are shaped much more by indirect than direct costs, since direct health care costs are effectively covered by health insurance' (Wörz 2011:20).

The East German health care system 1945–90

Following the fall of the Nazi regime in 1945, Germany was divided into two formally independent countries that were effectively under the jurisdiction of two distinct political and economic blocs. The Western bloc represented the wartime Allies, but in practice was dominated by the geo-political interests of the USA, and to a much lesser extent by Britain and France. The Eastern bloc was constituted by the newly established post-war Communist regimes in Eastern Europe but effectively dominated by the geo-political interests of the Soviet Union. It was in this context that the *Deutsche Demokratische Republik* (DDR), also known in English as the German Democratic Republic (GDR) or colloquially as East Germany, developed its health and welfare system quite separately from that of West Germany.

By 1950, the East German health care system was effectively nationalised and placed under centralised state control following the Soviet model. Yet while the new health system reflected the formal political commitment to social equality and equity of provision, it also contained elements of the pre-war German SHI structures. In the new system, a small number of doctors continued to provide ambulatory care in single-handed practices, but the majority became state employees providing care within state-run community or workplace-based polyclinics. Although the pre-war structural division between ambulatory and hospital services was formally preserved, in practice these separate health care sectors as well as the full range of health professionals, including doctors, were often located on the same premises and together collaborated to improve patient care (Busse et al:2017;887).

Some independent hospitals, both private and not-for-profit, continued to exist, but these gradually decreased in number over time, so that by 1989, only 7% of all hospital beds were not state-managed. Certain aspects of the Bismarckian SHI funding model were retained, insurance contributions were now mandatory and universal, but rather than the hundreds of sickness schemes that existed before the war there were now just two in the DDR: one insurance scheme for workers and their families covering 89% of the population, and one provided cover for the remaining 11% which included members of agricultural cooperatives, artists, and people who were self-employed. The contribution rate was never increased after 1971, however, given the rising costs of health care this ultimately led onto a significant underfinancing of the system (Busse et al:2017;887). Community level health prevention services were also established in the 1950s and included maternity and child health care, as well as specialist care for people with common chronic diseases such as diabetes or psychiatric disorders.

By the 1970s, the lack of investment in the DDR economy led onto skill shortages and a failure to keep up with technological developments in the West. This contributed to a reduction in the effective functioning of the health system, and a gap in the rates of mortality and morbidity as compared to the BRD began to develop. This was despite the fact that over the two previous decades both countries had experienced parallel improvements in life expectancy and even a slight advantage for men in East Germany. By the late 1980s, the number of hospital admissions per capita was approximately 25% lower than in the BRD. In response, a National Health Conference was organised in the first week of November 1989, this committed the government to introduce fundamental health care reforms along with an increase in investment; a few days later the Berlin Wall fell (Busse et al:2017;887). Following Free elections in the DDR in the spring of 1990, the political parties that stood on a platform of fast-track reunification won by a significant margin. The newly elected government immediately adopted the Deutsche Mark and began the negotiations that led onto the unification of Germany later that year, on 3 October 1990.

Reunification and reform of the German health care system

Reunification required a modernising of the former DDR health and welfare systems which were effectively subsumed within the existing BRD structures; but this process came at a considerable cost. It became apparent that raising the standard of living within the East to match that of the West would require a massive injection of spending by the now unified German state. An initial support package of £81.3bn (2019 prices) was provided and designed to cover the first six years of unification, this included the transfer of capital and equipment. But the largest single component of this funding was in the form of indirect transfers to the citizens of the former DDR, via the now unified social security and health care systems. According to the most recent estimates, more than £2 trillion (2019 prices) was spent on the reunification project between 1990 and 2018 (Enenkel & Rösel:2022;5).

Following unification, the western part of Germany was able to maintain strong levels of economic performance growth, as the former BRD government had borrowed heavily from the financial markets in order to sustain growth and so fund the process of unification. However by 1992, the impact of a new economic recession had begun to reduce the rate of growth which was to remain low for the remainder of the decade. The failure to sustain economic growth is often attributed solely to the costs of unification, but the government's fiscal policy was also a major contributor. The costs of servicing the national debt combined with the expansion of the social security/protection system across the unified nation led onto an increase in SHI contribution rates, as well as to cuts in other public services over the course of the 1990s. This increase in SHI contribution costs was then exacerbated by rising levels of unemployment in the East, as the 'oversized West German manufacturing sector had no need for additional production sites in the *Neue Länder*' (Streek:2020;49). However, the cumulative impact of the fiscal tightening undertaken by the CDU government has in hindsight been seen as excessive and way beyond Germany's actual public borrowing requirements. Over the course of the 1990s into the new Millennium, fiscal austerity resulted in protracted national budget deficits, with long-term implications for the SHI funding of the health care system (Bibow:2001;4).

In attempting to understand why German state economic policy in the post-war years right up until the present day has chosen to prioritise fiscal management and to limit public borrowing over and above the funding requirements of the health and welfare system, it is essential to recognise the long shadow cast by the 1929 Wall Street stock market 'crash'. The subsequent collapse of national banking systems in Germany primarily arose from a financial over-speculation that had no basis in economic reality. The 'crash' led onto the Great Depression and mass unemployment in the 1930s, both in the USA and across Europe. In Germany the effects of this global financial meltdown were felt particularly acutely in an economy that was still attempting to recover from the experience of hyperinflation in the previous decade. This hyperinflation itself resulted from the impact of military defeat in the First World War and the crippling financial reparations payments subsequently imposed on Germany. The Wall Street banking crash led on to the withdrawal of US loans that had been made to the German Weimer Government, this further set back an already weakened economy. Historians have traditionally argued that it was these economic factors that resulted in the social conditions that led onto the rise of the Nazi Regime in 1933, although today that perspective is rather more nuanced. Nevertheless, this historical memory of debt and economic depression remains strong in contemporary Germany. Drawing on survey data, Haffert et al (2021) found that many Germans could not clearly distinguish between the history of hyperinflation and that of the Great Depression, conceiving the two events, with a decade between them, as one and the same thing. About half of the survey participants also thought of the post-1929 Great Depression as a period of high inflation, whereas fewer than 5% knew that it was, in fact, a period of deflation (Galofré-Vilà:2021).

In post-war Germany, this economic history and its particular national interpretation have shaped the fiscal policies of CDU governments from the early 1950s up until reunification and beyond. Tight state control over public borrowing became an economic orthodoxy in West Germany and was given its own distinctive label, 'ordoliberalism'. Ordoliberalism sought to establish a legal and ethico-political framework (*Rahmenordnung*) for government to act to regulate markets to ensure that actual economic outcomes 'approximate the theoretical outcome in a perfectly competitive market' (Dullien & Guérot:2012). Ordoliberalism can be contrasted with the attempt to impose economic neoliberalism in Britain in the 1980s. While the CDU's position on social issues was always been broadly similar to that of the British Conservative Party, in economic matters it never embraced the Hayekian ideology of the small state and unregulated markets that became a key feature of Conservative governments from the 1980s onwards. As Bob Jessop has noted in his comparison of these two contrasting economic orthodoxies: 'One has a principled commitment, or at least a principled aspiration, to create an ordered society and reduce crisis tendencies; the other involves a consciously disruptive process that sees profitable opportunities in crisis and may create them' (Jessop:2019;2). Germany being an example of the former, and the UK the latter.

This 'principled commitment' to maintain price stability and economic competitiveness while at the same time attempting to manage the social and financial consequences of unification, inevitably, impacted on the financial sustainability of the German health care system by the early 1990s. At the same time, the German health system was also beginning to face the challenges now experienced by nearly all HIC countries, that of the rising costs of an ageing population, new medical technology, and increasing demands for high quality and responsive health care. These factors combined to produce recurrent annual deficits in health care financing, even as SHI schemes increased the level of individual and employer contribution rates. This predicament brought about the first significant calls for health system reform in Germany, focusing on the need to reduce costs and improve the efficiency of the service. This same appeal to fiscal rationality was also foremost in the Thatcher reforms in the NHS that were being implemented around the time, albeit in a different fiscal policy context.

The first post-unification reforms to the structure of the German health system were introduced in 1993. These changes were seen to mark: '(T)he most important paradigm shift in the history of statutory health insurance, since it not only eliminated the century-old occupational classification and the privileges that white-collar workers had compared with blue-collar workers, but also provided a new regulatory basis for competition among sickness funds and contracts between sickness funds and providers' (Knieps et al:2015, cited in Busse et al:2017;887). The thinking behind this shift in policy was to open up a new competitive market between sickness insurance schemes, and so promote a process of merger that in theory would reduce costs and improve efficiency. This proved to be the case, and by 2015 the number of funding schemes had been reduced by 70%, fundamentally changing the structure of the SHI system. Where once membership of an SHI scheme carried the political and social connotations that linked directly to the traditions of social solidarity in Germany, 'the member (of a social insurance scheme) is now more likely to be treated as a customer' (Busse et al:2017;889).

CDU-led coalition governments and the post-2005 health system reforms

In a period that stretching from 2005 until late 2021, Angela Merkel presided as Chancellor over four separate CDU-led coalition governments. All were marked by a determination to give primacy to limiting the country's financial deficit through the achievement of monetary stability. This was seen as crucial to maintaining Germany's competitive advantage in the global marketplace as an export-led economy. While, Merkel's leadership was not slavishly beholden to ordoliberal economic orthodoxy, her governments nevertheless sought to embed market competition in 'formally institutionalised, political forms of solidarity', replacing those traditional forms social solidarity central to the funding of German health and social protection systems (Streek:2020;57).

The focus of health policy in the post-2005 period was to achieve a measure of central control over costs through the introduction of the mechanism of competition between schemes, and a range of 'efficiency-enhancing policies'. New requirements for both internal and external quality control in health service provision were introduced. These encompassed structural, as well as process- and outcome-related dimensions of performance-management; particularly in relation to improvements in hospital inpatient services. In 2007, the first CDU-SPD coalition government (2005–09) enacted legislation that was self-explanatory given in its title, *Act to Strengthen Competition in Statutory Health Insurance*. Competition between SHI schemes was to be facilitated not by means of an 'internal market mechanism', as had been the case in the UK in the 1990s, but through the introduction of new regulatory mechanisms covering provision across the whole country.

Perhaps surprisingly, it was only in 2009 that universal SHI coverage (either through statutory health insurance or in private health insurance) was achieved. This development included a uniform minimum SHI contribution rate for the first time, while also offering a choice of tariffs (a feature previously reserved for private health insurance companies). The second CDU-Liberal Coalition government (2009–13) introduced further legislative change to promote health care provider competition, hoping that this would contain the costs of insurance scheme funding. In 2014, further regulations governing the contribution rates paid into SHI funds were introduced by the third CDU-SPD Coalition government (2013–17). The SHI schemes were now to be allowed to charge an additional rate on top of the uniform rate, to be paid by the policyholder only. However, with the Federal states having effective jurisdiction over both the SHI payers and the health care provider institutions located regionally, there were limits to just how far these reforms to the SHI contribution system could improve the efficiency of the health system as a national whole.

The third CDU-led Coalition government also introduced the *Hospital Structure Reform Act* in 2016. The importance of this legislation lay in the fact that it was an attempt to reform the inpatient sector of the health system through the introduction of more stringent quality assurance and efficiency measures. The chosen instrument of reform was an arms-length body, the independent Institute for Quality Assurance and Transparency in Healthcare (*Institut für Qualitätssicherung und Transparenz im Gesundheitswesen*) or IQTiG. The IQTiG had been established in 2009 as an advisory body to the Federal Joint Committee (*Gemeinsamer Bundesausschuss* – FJS), the central decision-making body responsible for the governance of health care provision across Germany. Its specific role being to provide evidence-based evaluations of cost benefits of services defined in terms of potential improvements in clinical outcomes (Blümel et al:2014). This was a similar arms-length role to that played by NICE within the NHS. Both bodies utilised similar assessment methodologies in order to arrive at their respective recommendations regarding new medical technologies, pharmaceuticals, and other clinical interventions. The main difference was that the IQTiG restricted itself to the clinical evidence alone, whereas NICE has the remit to apply the additional measure of 'cost-effectiveness', so is a more patient-outcome orientated assessment process (Ivandic:2014).

The 2016 legislation now gave the IQTiG a set of system-wide responsibilities. This ALB was now charged with developing national indicators for quality-based hospital planning, including the re-examination of contracts between sickness funds and hospitals, as well as the assessment of the potential of pay-for-performance in hospitals. This shift in focus to the enactment of rigorous quality assurance inspection reflected the limited room for manoeuvre that was available to the German central state in determining the direction and costs of health care; SHI as the key funding mechanism for health care provision not being under the direct control of

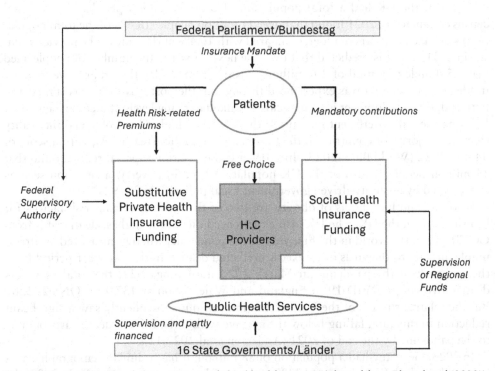

Figure 7.3 Organisational chart – German federal health system (Adapted from Blümel et al (2020)).

the central state. The Basic Law constitutional separation of roles as between the German state government and the 16 federal governments continues to be reflected in the existence of an array of governance relationships that pertain between private and SHI schemes, as well as between health care providers and purchasers in the different regional states.

The complex decentralised organisational relationships that characterise the governance and funding of the German health care system as they existed in 2020, are set out in a simplified schema in Figure 7.3. Health care providers are divided into three main sectors: hospitals, ambulatory or outpatient care,[11] and long-term care. The large number of SHI schemes includes some 106 Sickness Funds and 105 Long-term care Funds. While Substitutive Private Health Insurance (PHI) schemes include some 42 private insurance companies, as well as 42 long-term care private insurance companies. PHI now become available as a substitute for SHI to the self-employed, those above a set high-income threshold, as well as permanent public employees.

A fourth CDU-SPD coalition government was elected to office in 2018 under the Chancellorship of Angela Merkel and remained in power until she finally stepped down from office in October 2021. This is a suitable historical point at which to end this historical-institutional analysis of the development of health care provision in Germany.

A brief outline of population health status in the UK and Germany

Prior to commencing a comparative analysis of the performance of the UK and German health care systems, it is useful to undertake a brief outline of the current demography and health status of both populations.

In 2023, the UK had a total population of over 68 million people. The national census conducted in 2021 found that over 11 million people (18.6% of the total population) were aged 65 years or older, compared with 16.4% at the time of the previous census in 2011, and it is predicted that over the next 25 years, the number of people aged over 85 double to a total of 2.6 million (ONS:2022a). Today the progressive increase in life expectancy that was experienced throughout the post-war years has stalled and flattened, this development is seen as closely linked to rising levels of income inequality. Utilising the Gini coefficient measure,[12] the UK has a higher level of social inequality than the majority of countries in the European Economic Area (EEA), with a score of 34.4 in 2022 (World Bank:2023). In 2019, a United Nations Special report found that 14 million people, a fifth of the UK population lived in poverty, a situation seen as exacerbated by austerity-driven government fiscal policy (UN:2019).

Smoking and high levels of obesity are two of the most significant risk factors for health status in the UK. The UK also experienced one of the highest death rates from COVID-19 in the world in the first year of the pandemic, whether measured as attributable directly to the virus or as excess predicted deaths. In the two-year period from the outbreak of the pandemic in March 2020 until June 2022, the total of excess deaths involving COVID-19 in England and Wales stood at 137,000 (ONS:2022b). But the relative success of the UK vaccination roll-out subsequently saw a significant reduction in this rate, falling below the average within the EEA of deaths attributable to the pandemic by the end of 2021 (Anderson et al:2022;12).

In 2023, Germany had a population of 88 million. It has a similar demographic ageing profile to the UK, with around 22% of the population over the age of 65. In 2022, the

German economy was one of the most robust in the EEA, reflected in a per capita income of US$58.700, compared to US $49,000 in the UK, and an average of US$48,900 across the EU 27 member countries (OECD:2023). However, since 2022 the economy has stagnated and long-term growth prospects are limited. This development primarily results from the structural adjustment process now occurring in the key manufacturing sector in response to '(D)ecarboniztion, digitlization, and demographic change – alongside stronger competition with companies from China' (IFO Institute:2024).

Germany's Gini coefficient score remains slightly lower than that of the UK at 32.0 (World Bank:2023), nevertheless, income inequalities have been on the increase for more than a decade, and this has led in turn to widening inequalities in health outcome. At the point of reunification in 1990 there were significant differences in life expectancy between the West and East of Germany, and in the intervening 30 years, these differences have narrowed but not closed (Blümel:2020;9). Life expectancy fell for the first time between 2019 and 2022, reflective of the impact of the COVID-19 pandemic that accounted for over 1 million excess deaths. Mortality rates have since returned to average EU levels, these stand at 80.7 years of age for the population as a whole, with men living shorter lives than women by an average of 5 years. Germany has a similar profile of chronic disease to the UK. Cancers (at 22%) and heart disease (at 33%) are linked to the cause of approximately 55% of deaths, both disease conditions are associated with above average EU rates for smoking and alcohol consumption, as well as high fat diets and sedentary lifestyles. Some 18% of the German population have experienced a mental health condition, again slightly higher than the EU average (OECD/European Health Observatory:2023;3–6).

****

A comparative analysis of the German and UK health care systems

This comparative performance analysis of the UK and German health systems draws upon an assessment framework first developed by Claus Wendt (2009). The primary reason for adopting Wendt's analytical approach is that it was explicitly designed as a dedicated tool for the assessment of health systems within European welfare states. Wendt's (2009) framework is largely process-orientated, and its seven evaluative categories are primarily focused on regulation, provision, and financing and funding of health care systems with universal access.[13]

Note: The application of Wendt's framework does not imply that the comparative analysis framework utilised to compare Kenya and Ghana in the previous chapter should be restricted only to the analysis of LIDC health systems. But rather, and consistent with the position that historical and institutional context is key to understanding the development and performance of health systems, a one-size-fits-all approach to comparative performance analysis can be overly reductive.

1. Health expenditure

The UK: Total health expenditure (THE) as a percentage share of GDP was 10.9% in 2023, a slight decrease from 11.1% in 2021 reflecting the additional costs of the COVID-19 pandemic (ONS:2024). This expenditure accounts for nearly a fifth of all public spending in the UK, and over 30% of spending on public services (not including national debt interest and transfers such as social security benefits). Since the founding of the NHS in 1948, state spending on health care has grown at an average rate of 3.7% a year (Charlesworth & Johnson:2018), but with significant variation at different historical periods (see Figure 7.1). Between 1996 and 2009, during a period of economic growth and expansion, public spending on health grew at an average real term increase of 5.3% per year (ONS:2023), but averaged just a 1.4% real terms increase per year since the imposition of government fiscal austerity in 2009. Since 2005 when it represented 81% of THE, the proportion of public spending on health has remained largely unchanged, in 2023 it constituted 81.9% of THE (ONS:2024). Funding is primarily targeted towards secondary care services to the long-term detriment of spending on public health and social care.

Germany: Health expenditure as a percentage share of GDP in Germany was 11.7% in 2019, the year prior to the increased expenditure required for the containment of the COVID-19 pandemic. This equates to a higher level of per capita spending than in almost all other European countries. However, in comparison to systems funded by direct taxation such as the UK, this relatively high level of spending also reflects the additional costs of operating a decentralised SHI funding system. Each of the 105 sickness funds collect the mandatory SHI contributions, these are then transferred into a central reallocation known as the *Gesundheitsfonds*, which in turn is responsible for pooling and reallocating these revenues according to a risk-adjustment mechanism (Blümel et al:2020;76). This process involves a significant bureaucratic input with associated costs, whereas in the centralised NHS only 2% of health expenditure is spent on administration (OECD:2022b).

2. Private-public financing mix

The UK: Public spending on health is represented almost entirely by the funding of the NHS (82%), financed through direct taxation and national insurance payments. The 18% of THE that represents non-government financial sources includes (i) Private or 'Voluntary' health insurance. (ii) Enterprise financing – covering health care activity funded by organisations (primarily employers) outside of an insurance scheme, such as occupational health care. (iii) Out-of-pocket (OOP) expenditure – including client contributions for local authority and NHS-provided services and prescription charges. (iv) Charitable financing – referred to as-profit institutions, and covering expenditure funded through voluntary donations, grants, and investment income.

Critical assessments of the history of market reforms to the NHS consistently identify a process of 'creeping privatisation' (Kings Fund:2018), while the long-term impact of austerity budgets from 2009 onwards has seen a year-on-year increase in waiting times for treatment. This underinvestment in the NHS has seen a rise in the outsourcing of elective procedures to the private sector, which equated to 10% of all elective procedures in 2023, a 29% increase in a period of just four years (IHPN:2024). An increasing number of patients are now self-paying so they can avoid the uncertainties of being on an NHS waiting list, and receive their necessary treatment in the private sector. The numbers of self-payers and those signing up for Private Medical Insurance schemes for the first time rose 23% from pre-COVID-19 to the end of 2023 (IHPN:2024).

Germany: Traditionally in Germany, there is a close relationship of co-existence between SHI and private health insurance funding of health care that was consciously promoted by the government even prior to unification in 1989. However, the attempt to facilitate widening popular participation in PHI schemes through reforms to the system of funding stalled following the decision in 2009 to make SHI payments mandatory. The effective rowing back on the promotion of PHI also reflects the new central regulatory role of the IQTiG, whose mission is to ensure that health expenditure is effectively linked to provider performance and value-for-money outcomes. In a society with an increasingly ageing population with long-term health needs, promoting the uptake of private provision is now recognised as resulting in a widening of the gap in health care equity. The share of public spending as a percentage of THE has gradually increased from 78.2% in 2000 to 84.6% in 2008 (WHO:2023). As Blümel et al (2020;71) have pointed out, this apparent increase in the proportion of public spending on health is largely explained by the introduction of mandatory SHI, and the ending of voluntary coverage for some employment groups.

3. Privatisation of risk

The UK: Individual out-of-pocket (OOP) payments represent the largest single element of non-government health spending. Between 1997 and 2018, individual OOP payments grew in real terms by an average annual rate of 3.3%, and voluntary PHI schemes grew by an average rate of 2.6%. In 2022, OOP payments totalled £40.4 billion, representing 13.8% of the £292 billion UK THE, a 3% real terms increase from the previous year (ONS:2024). The largest single item of OOP spending was on medical goods (predominantly pharmaceuticals, but also hearing aids and eyewear), and the remainder was spent on rehabilitative and long-term care.

Germany: Since the 2009, all German residents have been legally required to have health insurance either in SHI (87%) or substitutive PHI (11%); the remaining 2% are in the military that are covered by special insurance programmes. In 2020, the opt-out threshold (changes annually) for SHI was set at an individual income of €62.5K, so PHI is only a voluntary option for a small minority of the population. As in the UK, there is no requirement for residents to take on these additional personal insurance payments, as benefits are the same for all in the SHI universal provision system. There is a comparatively low degree of health cost sharing, with individual OOP representing 12.3% of THE in 2018 (comparable to the UK level). This OOP spending is primarily linked to medical goods, some ambulatory or outpatient services, but with the largest proportion spent on co-payment costs for inpatient stays (Blümel et al:2020;85).

4. Health service provision

The UK: The proportion of national spending allocated to the provision of primary preventive services, secondary care provision, as well as tertiary care services, is a broad reflection of the relative priority accorded by government to each sector. From a health economics perspective, provision represents the 'supply' side of a health care system and includes the health workforce with its particular skill mix, the range and number of health care facilities including hospital beds, and the accessibility of primary care services to local populations. The NHS is typical of many health care systems in HICs in disproportionally resourcing hospital-based secondary care. Spending on primacy care services represented just 8% of the UK government health care budget in 2021–22, while spending on long-term tertiary care represented just 14.5% (BMA:2023/ONS:2023). It should also be noted that the NHS provision of long-term beds does not constitute social care provision; this remains the statutory responsibility of local government social services departments in England and Wales.

Despite the disproportionate level of resources allocated to secondary care, the overall number of NHS hospital beds for acute care management is proportionately lower than in most other high-income health care systems. The number of beds decreased from 4.1 to 2.5 beds per 1,000 population during the period 2000–18. In part this reflects the historical trend of reducing the length of stay in hospital resulting from improvement in clinical management, including an increase in day surgery units. But this is a trend that has been more marked in the UK than elsewhere. The unforeseen consequences of this policy were apparent during the COVID-19 pandemic when the demand for acute care rose dramatically and could not be met by the existing facilities (Anderson et al:2022;87).

In terms of the NHS workforce in England,[14] as of March 2024, full-time equivalent (FTE) staff numbers were 1,345,057, representing a headcount of 1,506,043 individual staff[15] (NHS Digital:2024a). This represents a higher proportional increase over the period of a decade (1,203,519 FTE in June 2014) than the real term increase in state health spending over the same period. Professionally qualified clinical frontline staff numbered 711,117 FTE, this represents a 5.8% increase over the period of one year to March 2023, but proportionate to the 5.1% increase in all NHS staff groups over the same period. The number of professionally qualified clinical staff constituted 52.9% of the total NHS workforce in March 2024 (NHS Digital:2024a). Yet there remain significant numbers of vacancies for all clinical professional's, with a 6% vacancy rate for doctors and 7.5% for nursing staff in England at the end of the fourth quarter in 2023–24 (NHS Digital:2024b). This high vacancy rate for clinical staff reflects a range of factors, but primarily a combination of relatively low-pay compared to the private health sector, and exponentially increasing workloads not limited to the two-year period during which the COVID-19 pandemic saw significant admissions to hospital. This increase in staff workload has led to long-term high levels of stress and illness. In 2023 and in early 2024, there were an unprecedented number of strikes days over low pay and working conditions involving both nursing staff and doctors that sought to improve low pay and working conditions.

Germany: The trend towards reducing beds for acute care in large-scale hospitals has been on-going in the health system for some time, yet Germany has maintained a ratio of 6.02 beds per 1,000 population (as per 2017), the second highest in the European Union. It should be noted though, that the average bed-occupancy rate across the country is less than 80%, which in turn impacts on the economic viability of private provider services. By comparison, prior to the COVID-19 epidemic, bed-occupancy rate in the NHS was running at 90.2% – BMA:2022). Despite the decrease in acute beds, the high overall numbers of beds reflect an institutional shift towards the provision of more psychiatric beds as well as an increase in long-term care beds in nursing and residential accommodation, which have together increased by 40% since 2000 (Eurostat:2020).

The decentralised structure of the German health care system has undoubtedly resulted in a fragmentation of provision across the country, and although a dense network of hospitals exists in Germany meaning that, 'virtually everyone can reach an acute care hospital by car within 30 minutes … (but) discrepancies persist between the (16 regional) states, as the latter are responsible for capital investment and hospital planning' (Blümel et al:2020;109). The regional states have the responsibility for financing capital investment in hospital and clinic facilities, while day-to-day running costs are funded through the various SHI sickness funds, PHI companies, and individual co-payments. This has produced a situation, where for example the State of Hamburg spends three times as much as the State of Saxony-Anhalt per bed, €9304 as against €3038 in 2017 (Blümel et al:2020;118).

These marked regional inequities would be unsustainable within a centralised financing system such as the NHS.

The German health system workforce is organised on the same decentralised basis as the institutional infrastructure, but centralised governance mechanisms for planning human resources are largely absent. For example, the number of places available for the academic training of health professionals is determined by individual universities, not the Federal government nor the regional states. Yet the regional states have the responsibility for regulating and financing clinical education, as well as registering and supervising professionals (Blümel et al:2020;122). In the UK, the majority of these responsibilities are centralised through the Department of Health and Social Care or its devolved ALBs. In 2020, Germany had the 6th highest proportion of nurses and doctors per 100,000 population in Western Europe, whereas the UK was in 17th position (WHO Regional Office for Europe:2022). Yet despite these high ratios, the German system is currently experiencing a shortage of health professionals in critical areas similar to that found in the UK and for many of the same reasons.

Not dissimilar to the UK, the different sectors of health care (primary or out-patient ambulatory care; in-patient hospital-based care; and public health) are separated in the German system. This separation is not only in terms of organisational structure and regulatory oversight, but also in terms of planning and financing. This results in the fragmentation previously described, in relation to the coordination, quality assurance, as well as efficiency of the health service (Blümel et al:2020;139).

5. Entitlement to health care

The UK: The basis of entitlement within the system of universal provision is one of health or clinical need rather than citizenship per se. Primary care services are free of charge to all those who are registered as a local patient, or as a temporary patient if someone is living in the area for more than 24 hours and less than 3 months. The available services include community-based professionals such as GPs, practice nurses, and midwives, as well as dentists, pharmacists, optometrists, and other specialised community services. Entitlement to secondary care services is a residence-based one, meaning that access to free health care is on the basis of living lawfully in the UK on a properly settled basis (no requirement to be a UK citizen). This measure of entitlement is known as 'ordinary residence'. Individuals who are not ordinarily resident in the UK may be required to pay for their care, but some services and some individuals are exempt. Prior to Brexit, all citizens of the EEA were able to access all NHS services free of charge, with reciprocal arrangements in place for UK nationals. Since formally leaving the EU on December 31, 2020, EEA nationals are now subject to the same rules as non-EEA nationals when accessing NHS services (Office for Health Improvement and Disparities:2023).

Germany: The German system is also structured on the basis of universal health provision funded through compulsory membership of an insurance-based system that is linked to income not health risk, with non-earning spouses and children insured free of charge. Insured patients are entitled to all therapeutic services, not only physician services but also those provided by allied health professionals such as speech therapists, physiotherapists, occupational therapists, etc. However, reimbursement of care provided by these allied health professionals is dependent on a referral being provided by a doctor. There is also free entitlement to all medical aids such as glasses, hearing aids, wheelchairs, etc, with individuals reimbursed the cost of the pharmaceuticals they require through their SHI schemes. However, there are certain population groups who remain at risk of not having health insurance despite the 2009 legislation.

6. Remuneration of doctors

The UK: This evaluative category is based on the reasonable assumption that the form of remuneration is a key indicator of whether there are sufficient 'incentives' for doctors to provide what is termed 'high volume' health care, the delivery of quality care for an increasing workload of patients.

In the NHS, all junior hospital doctors (which includes all medically qualified staff from Foundation level up to and including specialised senior staff) are salaried, but medical consultants constitute a separate category of medical staff and have their own contractual arrangements with the NHS. The Consultant contract (as negotiated between the Consultants Committee of the BMA and the NHS employers) offers pay supplements and a sliding scale of rewards additional to a basic NHS salary. Additionally, Consultants have the right to maintain their own private practice, but only after meeting their contractual working hours within the NHS. The ability of medical consultants to mix private and NHS work has existed since the inception of the NHS in 1946. Aneurin Bevin, the Minister of Health at the time, was famously quoted as saying he had 'stuffed their mouths with gold' in order to persuade the Consultants to agree to join the new NHS. However, as the terms of the national contract for Consultants have been re-negotiated over the years, the original mix of working hours in favour of the time spent working in the private sector has gradually been eroded. Today most Consultants spend the majority of their working time undertaking NHS work.

GPs working in primary care have also always enjoyed a distinct contractual status within the NHS, operating as 'independent contractors' while contractually tied to working exclusively for the NHS. GPs also have a separately negotiated contract which is agreed between its representative body, the General Practitioners Committee of the BMA, and NHS England. But unlike the Consultants, this contract is negotiated annually. In addition, there are monetary incentives for GP practices (not individual doctors) through the meeting of national targets for screening and treatment guidelines that are set within the Quality Outcomes Framework (QOF).

Germany: In 2019, according to the Federal Association of SHI Physicians, 44% of all active physicians in Germany worked in SHI-contracted ambulatory care, the majority being self-employed in solo practices. These physicians are reimbursed through the sickness schemes on a fee-for-service basis set at a regional, not a national uniform rate. But this situation has been subject to change in recent years. The numbers of physicians working as salaried members of staff in interdisciplinary primary care medical centres increased by 117% over the decade from 2009 to 2018; an admittedly from a very low base. At the same time, the total number of physicians in family medicine increased by 4% (Blümel et al:2020;151). Physicians providing specialised care in hospitals are primarily salaried employees. But more senior doctors are able to treat patients who are in-privately insured on a fee-for-service basis. In comparing the NHS and the German system, remuneration of physicians in the different health care sectors is on similar lines, even if the institutional structures of health care are quite distinct from one another.

7. Patient access

The UK: In the NHS, GPs in primary care settings are not only the first point of contact for patients, they are also the 'gatekeepers' for referrals onto specialist treatment in the secondary care sector. They therefore act as a key cost containment mechanism for the health system as a whole. However, the failure to recruit and retain sufficient GPs (as well as other primary care health professionals), to meet the increasing demand for primary care has led to increasing problems for patients in accessing primary care services when required. This has led onto the situation whereby hospital accident and emergency departments have now, by default, become a key entry point to the health care system as a whole. This has proven particularly problematic in terms of increasing waiting times for those who do require emergency or urgent care. Patient referral for secondary care is based on clinical need, but the many pressures on the system described above, have led to a significant increase in waiting times for routine care and delays to follow up.

In 2019 (prior to Brexit), the UK was identified as having one of the highest levels of unmet need for medical examination across all EU member countries (Eurostat:2019), however this unmet need is unevenly spread. Some 4.9% of those in the lowest income quintile requiring medical examination report unmet medical need, while the equivalent figure for the highest income quintile is just 3.3% (Anderson et al:2022;151). By way of comparison, the same data set identified Germany as having one of the lowest levels of unmet need for a medical examination in the EU, while at the same time having a similar difference to the UK as between low- and high-income population groups.

Germany: No compulsory gate-keeping system exists in the German health system; patients can freely choose any SHI-accredited doctor for whatever type of health care treatment they require, whether primary or specialist care. However, this absence of a gate-keeping system has led onto 'a fragmented and uncoordinated service provision' (Blümel et al:2020;154). Ambulatory or primary care has long been dominated by single-handed practice-based physicians, but more recently there has been a trend towards the development of greater cooperative between providers. This has facilitated the gradual adoption of structured patient pathways through the health system, broadly modelled on those that function within the NHS. Patients who enrol in this 'GP-centred model of care' agree to consult their GP before referral on for specialist care. This development remains a voluntary one, but in 2020, some 17,000 GPs participated in this care model, covering some 5.4 million insured individuals (Blümel et al:2020;154).

Regional disparities in accessing hospital in-patient care services still exist within the German health system; this is despite several reforms over the past decade. Policy developments to address regional inequity have included the provision of financial incentives to physicians to work in 'underserved area', and attempts to contain 'oversupply' in some regions by refusing licences for new ambulatory care physicians. Perhaps most significantly, the Federal government has attempted to limit some of the inequities that have arisen through decentralised health care provision through a commitment to promote needs-based planning (Blümel et al:2020;198).

Concluding comments: differences and commonalities

The main limitation of Wendt's (2009) seven evaluative performance categories that form the basis of this comparative outcomes analysis is that they marginalise the role played by health policy actors. These limitations were acknowledged by the author when he stated that: '(C)oncentrating not only on actors and institutions but also on out-comes may combine the strengths of different disciplines and is theoretically valuable, practically feasible, and policy relevant … Furthermore, healthcare systems themselves are the outcomes of health policy decisions, which demonstrates the inter-relationship between health policy actors and healthcare systems' (Marmor & Wendt:2012;18). This comparative analysis of the German and UK health systems has attempted to offset these limitations with the inclusion of a historical institutional analysis that does give due prominence to the key policy actors, both institutional and individual.

The material presented within this chapter in general points to the differences between these two health care systems as being less significant than their shared commonalities. The differences primarily flow from two key factors, the decentralised nature of the fed-eral structure of governance in Germany and its historical and cultural commitment to the SHI funding system. This is by comparison with the command-and-control structure of the health system in the UK (noting that strategic health decision-making in Scotland, Northern Ireland and Wales is devolved to their respective governments), as well as its direct taxation funding system. These institutional and structural differences has meant that the German health system requires higher levels of expenditure to achieve a comparative level of health outcomes because of its additional bureaucratic layers. In effect, there exists a diffused system of policy decision-making which has set significant challenges for the effec-tive governance of the German health system, particularly in ensuring the coherence and efficiency of equitable national provision. A recognition of these limitations is reflected in the more recent attempts to develop national oversight institutions for quality control and standard-setting. There is also a belated recognition that a vertical redistribution of Federal resources from richer to poorer *Länder*, in accordance with the constitutional require-ments, is necessary to ensure fiscal equity across the country (Greer et al:2023;14).

The necessity for the Federal government to take a more direct centralising role was particularly apparent during the COVID-19 pandemic, when the regional *Länder* were slow to initially react to limit the spread of the disease. Following a proposal by the Ministry of Health, a legislative amendment was made to the pre-existing *Prevention and Control of Infection Disease Act*. This allowed for a temporary transfer of powers to the Federal executive for one year in order to roll out a national pandemic plan admin-istered at national level. This enabled a national 'test-trace-isolate-support' strategy to be implemented, the supply of medications and vaccines to come through a centralised pur-chasing system, as well as to ensure the appropriate medical technologies and staff were in place across all the regions. The result was a significant drop in excess deaths as well as enabling a relative 'normalisation' to occur in school attendance and opening of services (Greer et al:2023;13). In the centralised UK system, after an initial slow and confused response on the part of government, the pre-existing national systems of procurement for vaccines as well as for the distribution of resources such as ITU beds, medical equip-ment and protective clothing ultimately proved to be effective in lowering excess deaths.

The vagaries of the processes associated with economic and financial globalisation present challenges for the funding and long-term fiscal planning for both systems, whether inside or outside of the European Union. Both countries have looked to the potential of the marketisation of health care provision as a solution to rising health costs, and both have found it wanting. More positively, there remains a shared history of a popular commitment to retaining the organising principles of equitable and uni-versal health coverage in both societies.

Notes

1 The Beveridge Report, its background and detailed recommendations was described in detail in Chapter 1.
2 This was the same fate that befell the Black Report into Inequalities in Health published the same year. These events are described in detail in Chapter 9.
3 Neoliberal economics and described in detail in Chapter 1.
4 The British economy was to go into recession yet again within less than two years, in 1991. This recession was linked to a global rise in interest rates following a US banking crisis (a pattern that was to repeat itself in 2008 but with much longer and deeper economic consequences), but was not anticipated by orthodox economists at the time.
5 The NPM and its legacy are discussed in detail in Chapter 3.
6 Arms-length bodies (ALBs) is a term that covers a wide variety of public sector institutions in the UK (currently there are approximately 300 operating within the UK). What ALBs have in common is their relative independence from central government ministerial control in fulfilling their roles and functions. But they remain ultimately accountable as publicly funded bodies to central government. They are not unique to the UK and exist in the majority of European states, including Germany.
7 The ongoing regulatory role of NICE, its technology assessment process, and its relationship with Big Pharma is discussed in detail in Chapter 10.
8 The principles and politics underpinning the governance and regulatory reforms of health systems were outlined in Chapter 3.
9 See Chapter 1 regarding the influence of Hayek on the development neo-liberal thinking.
10 This embargo was instigated as a consequence of the Arab-Israeli war of that year and was directed at the Western countries (including Britain and West Germany) who supported the Israel war fought against Egypt and Syria who were attempting to regain territory they had lost during their 1967 war with Israel.
11 What is termed 'ambulatory' care in many European health systems are walk-in medical services provided within the community. In the UK this services generally come under the heading of 'primary care services'.
12 The Gini coefficient is defined as 'the extent to which the distribution of income among individuals or households within an economy deviates from a perfectly equal distribution. With a Gini index score of 0 representing perfect equality, while an index of 100 implies perfect inequality' (World Bank:2023).
13 This framework is set out as Table 5.3 in Chapter 5 where its evaluative categories are described in outline.
14 The numbers do not include NHS staff working in Scotland, Wales, and Northern Ireland. These NHS staff are employed by the devolved ALBs respective to these three countries.
15 The NHS is now the largest single employer in England.

References

Anderson, P (2016) The heirs of Gramsci, *New Left Review*. no. 100.
Anderson, M, Pitchforth, E, Edwards, N, Alderwick, H, McGuire, A and Mossialos, E (2022) United Kingdom Health system review, *Health Systems in Transition*, vol. 24, no. 1. LSE Health/The Health Foundation/Nuffield Trust/European Observatory on Health Systems and Policies.
Bauernschuster, S, Driva, A and Hornung, E (2020) Bismarck's health insurance and the mortality decline, *Journal of the European Economic Association*, vol. 18, no. 5, 2561–2607.
Beveridge Report (1942) *Social Insurance and Allied Services*. Cmd 6404. London. HMSO.
Bibow, J (2001) The economic consequences of German unification. *Levy Institute Public Policy Brief No. 67*. Annandale-on-Hudson, NY. The Levy Economics Institute
Blümel, M, Panteli, D and van Ginneken, E (2014) Assuring quality of inpatient care in Germany: Existing and new approaches, *Eurohealth*, vol. 20, no. 3, 52–55.
Blümel, M, Spranger, A, Achstetter, K, Maresso, A and Busse, R (2020) Germany: Health system review, *Health Systems in Transition*, vol. 22, no. 6. Technische Universität Berlin/European Observatory on Health Systems and Policies.
BMA – British Medical Association (2022) *NHS Hospital Beds data analysis*. https://www.bma.org.uk/ (accessed 10/2022).

BMA – British Medical Association (2023) *Health Funding Data Analysis*. www.bma.org.uk (accessed 05/2023).

Busse, R, Blümel, M, Knieps, F and Bärnighausen, T (2017) Statutory health insurance in Germany: a health system shaped by 135 years of solidarity, self-governance, and competition, *The Lancet*, vol. 390, 882–897.

Carter, R (2020) After the long boom: the reconfiguration of work and labour in the public sector, *Historical Studies in Labour Relations*, vol. 41, no. 1, 137–168.

Charlesworth, A and Johnson, P (2018) *Securing the Future: Funding Health and Social Care to the 2030s*. London. Institute of Fiscal Studies/The Health Foundation.

Department of Health (1997) *The New NHS: Modern, Dependable*. Cm 3807. London. HMSO.

Dullien, S and Guérot, U (2012) *The long shadow of ordoliberalism: Germany's approach to the euro crisis*. European Council on Foreign Relations – Policy Brief. https://ecfr.eu (accessed 06/23).

Enenkel, K and Rösel, F (2022) *German reunification: lessons from the German approach to closing regional economic divides*. economy2030.resolutionfoundation.org (accessed 06/2023).

Eurostat (2019) *Unmet need for medical examination (due to cost, waiting time, or travel distance) by income quintile*. https://ec.europa.eu/eurostat/statistics-explained/index.php?title=Unmet_health_care_needs_statistics (accessed 10/2020).

Eurostat (2020) Long-term care beds in nursing and residential facilities. https://ec.europa.eu/eurostat/en/data/database (accessed 04/2023).

Evans, R (2024) Not so special, *London Review of Books*, vol. 46, no. 5, 17–18.

Fraser, D (1973) *The Evolution of the British Welfare State*. Basingstoke. Macmillan Press.

Galofré-Vilà, G (2021) *Debunking the idea that interwar hyperinflation in Germany led to the rise of the Nazi Party*. https://blogs.lse.ac.uk. October 19, 2021.

Greener, I and Powell, M (2021) Bevan, Beveridge and institutional change in the UK welfare state, *Social Policy and Administration*, vol. 56, no. 2, 271–283.

Greer, S, Dubin, K, Falkenbach, M, Jarman, H and Trump, B (2023) Alignment and authority: federalism, social policy, and the COVID-19 response, *Health Policy*, vol. 127, 12–18.

Haffert, L, Redecker, N and Rommel, T (2021) Misremembering Weimar: hyperinflation, the great depression, and German collective economic memory, *Economics and Politics*, vol. 33, no. 3, 664–686.

Ham, C (1992) *Health Policy in Britain* (2nd Ed). Basingstoke. Macmillan.

Health and Care Act (2022) https://legislation.gov.uk/ukpga/2022/31/contents (accessed 01/2023).

Health and Social Care Act (2012) https://legislation.gov.uk/ukpga/2012/7/contents (accessed 01/2023).

Health Foundation (2015) *How Funding for the NHS has changed over a rolling ten year period*. www.health.org.uk (accessed 07/2022).

Hockerts, H (1981) 'German Post-war social policies against the background of the Beveridge Plan' in Mommsen, W (ed) *The Emergence of the Welfare State in Britain and Germany 1850–1950*. London. Croom Helm, pp 315–341.

House of Commons Health Select Committee (2010) *Commissioning – Fourth Report*. London. Stationary Office.

IFO Institute (2024) *German economy in transition – Weak momentum, low potential growth*. The Joint Economic Forecast Project group. https://ifo.de (accessed 09/2024)

IHPN – Independent Healthcare Providers Network (2024) *Going Private: A Briefing on private Primary care* (February 8, 2024). https://Ihpn.org.uk (accessed 03/24).

Ivandic, V (2014) Requirements for benefit assessment in Germany and England: overview and comparison, *Health Economics Review*, no. 4:12.

Jessop, B (2019) Ordoliberalism and neoliberalization: governing through order or disorder, *Critical Sociology*, vol. 45, no. 7/8, 967–981.

Kings Fund (2018) *Is the NHS being Privatised?* www.kingsfund.org.uk (accessed 12/2022).

Kings Fund (2022) *Integrated Care Systems Explained*. www.kingsfund.org.uk (accessed 12/2023).

Klein, R (1995) *The New Politics of the NHS* (3rd Ed). London. Longman.

Klein, R (2001) *The New Politics of the NHS* (4th Ed). Harlow. Pearson.

Knieps, F and Reiners, H (2015) *Gesundheitsreformen in Deutschland: Geschichte-Intentionen-Kontroversen*. Bern. Verlag Hans Huber.

Lloyd, T (2015) *Funding Overview – Historical Trends in the UK*. London. The Health Foundation.

Marmor, T and Wendt, C (2012) Conceptual frameworks for comparing healthcare politics and policy, *Health Policy*, vol. 107, 11–20.

Merrison Committee Report (1979) *The Royal Commission of the National Health Service*. London. Stationary Office.

Moran, M (1999) *Governing the Health Care State*. Manchester. Manchester University Press.

NHS Digital (2024a) *NHS Workforce Statistics – March 2024*. https://digital.nhs.uk/data-and-information/publications/statistical/nhs-workforce-statistics (accessed 06/2024).

NHS Digital (2024b) *NHS Vacancy Statistics England, April 2015–March 2024*. https://digital.nhs.uk/data-and-information/publications/statistical/nhs-vacancies-survey/ (accessed 06/2024).

NHS England (2014) *Five Year Forward View*. London. NHS.

OECD (2022) *Health Statistics*. https://data.oecd.org/health.htm (accessed 12/2022).

OECD (2023) *Level of GDP per Capita & Productivity*. https://stats.oecd.org (accessed 10/2023).

OECD/European Observatory on Health Systems and Policies European Commission (2023) *Germany Country Health Profile 2023 – State of Health in the EU*. Paris. OECD Publishing.

Office for Health Improvement and Disparitie (2023) *NHS Entitlements: Migrant Health Guide*. https://www.gov.uk/guidance/nhs-entitlements-migrant-health-guide#immigration-health (accessed 05/2023).

Office of National Statistics (2015) *Employment and the Labour Market – An overview*. www.ons.gov.uk (accessed 10/2023).

Office of National Statistics (2022a) *Voices of Our Ageing Population: Living Longer Lives*. www.ons.gov.uk (accessed 06/2023).

Office of National Statistics (2022b). *Excess deaths in England and Wales: March 2020-June 2022*. www.ons.gov.uk (accessed 06/2023).

Office of National Statistics (2023) *Health Care Expenditure. UK Health Accounts: 2022*. www.ons.gov.uk (accessed 11/2023).

Office of National Statistics (2024) *Health Care Expenditure. UK Health Accounts: 2023*. www.ons.gov.uk (accessed 07/2024).

Paton, C (2006) *New Labour's State of Health; Political Economy, Public Policy and the NHS*. Aldershot. Ashgate.

Paton, C (2014) *At what cost? Paying the price for the market in the English NHS*. Centre for Health and the Public Interest (CHPI).

Pollitt, C (1995) Justification by works or faith? Evaluating the new public management, *Evaluation*, vol. 1, no. 2, 133–154.

Rosenhaft, E (1994) 'The historical development of German Social Policy' in Clasen, J and Freeman, R (eds) *Social Policy in Germany*. London. Harvester Wheatsheaf, pp 21–41.

Speed, E and Gabe, J (2020) The reform of the English NHS: professional dominance, counter-vailing powers and the buyers revolt, *Social Theory and Health*, vol. 18, 33–49.

Streek, W (2020) *Critical Encounters*. London. Verso.

Thelen, K (1999) Historical institutionalism in comparative politics, *Annual Review of Political Science*, vol. 2, 369–404.

United Nations (2019) *Visit to the UK – Report of the Special Rapporteur on extreme poverty and human rights*. https://un.org (accessed 03/2023).

Webster, C (2002) *The National Health Service: A Political History* (2nd Ed). Oxford. Oxford University Press.

Wendt, C (2009) Mapping European healthcare systems: a comparative analysis, *Journal of European Social Policy*, vol. 19, no. 5, 432–445.

World Bank (2022) *GDP growth (annual %) United Kingdom*. http://data.worldbank.org (accessed 02/2023).

World Bank (2023) *Gini Index UK and Germany*. https://data.worldbank.org (accessed 04/2023).

World Health Organisation (2023) *Global Health Expenditure Database*. https://apps.who.int/nha/database/Home/Index/en (accessed 01/2023).

World Health Organisation, Regional Office for Europe (2022) *European Health for All Database.* https://gateway.euro.who.int/en/datasets/european-health-for-all-database/ (accessed 02/2023).

Wörz, M (2011) Financial Consequences of Falling Ill: Changes in the German Health Insurance System since the 1980s. *WZB Discussion Paper, No. SP I 2011–209.* Wissenschaftszentrum Berlin für Sozialforschung (WZB), Berlin.

Zöllner, D (1982) 'Germany' in Köhler, H, Zacher, H and Partington, M (eds) *The Evolution of Social Insurance 1881–1981.* London. Pinter.

Challenges for Health Policy and Health Systems

Introduction to Section III

The third section of this book focuses attention on three challenges now facing health systems, each with significant implications for the direction of health policy now and in the future. Each of these challenges are posed as questions:

- How do societies in high-income countries (HICs) meet the increasing demand for health and social care following the demographic shift towards ageing populations?
- Public health strategies are uniformly acknowledged to be the most effective means of addressing the widening of social inequalities in health outcome in populations across the globe, yet why is it the case that public investment in public health remains low in comparison with secondary hospital-based clinical care in many health care systems?
- How does strategic health policy decision-making incorporate the clinical advances made possible by the evolving science of human genomics and the emergent diagnostic and treatment technologies known as 'precision medicine', while at the same time continuing to meet the significant population health 'burden' of chronic illness and disability?

****

The first challenge arises from the demographic shift within the majority of HIC's that has in turn led onto an inexorable rise in demand for long-term health and care services. This increase in demand now threatens to overwhelm the existing structures of health and social care in many countries. The use of statistical measures such as the 'old-age dependency ratio' focus attention on how government can best balance the requirements of the economy and ensure the robustness of public finances, as the proportion of those participating in the workforce begins to shrink. But focusing exclusively on the economic and fiscal consequences of an increasingly ageing population, important as this undoubtedly is, frequently distracts from the necessity of engaging with the known inadequacies of the existing structures of health and long-term social care provision. Addressing the need to construct a fully integrated care service, where social care support is provided on the same equitable basis as health care, is an issue

DOI: 10.4324/9781003564249-11

that continues to be eschewed in health policy-making. There being little evidence of significant progress in widening social care provision across all European welfare states in recent years.

The second challenge concerns the continuing existence of social inequalities in health outcome. Such inequalities are not a natural phenomenon, their continuing existence in rich and poor countries alike across the globe does not constitute some form of 'normal distribution' pattern of biological or genetic difference. Social differences in health outcomes are not inevitable or unavoidable; they reflect material differences between social groups over the course of a lifetime. Social inequalities (not the difference with 'social inequities'[1]) stem from structured social divisions and as such directly impact on the 'life chances' (including health outcomes) of large sections of the population. The primary social divisions relate to socio-economic class and income, but they also exist in terms of gender and ethnic differences. Increasingly there is a belated recognition that social inequalities are manifested in higher levels of obesity, increases in stress-related heart disease and other chronic conditions, deteriorating levels of mental health, and intensified vulnerability to infectious disease epidemics. The question then arises as to whether inequalities in health outcome are potentially amenable if there was a higher level of public investment in integrated public health programmes than is currently the case? The reality is that while the evidence points incontrovertibly to the effectiveness of 'upstream' interventions, national health policy and practice have frequently marginalised preventative health initiatives. As noted by the WHO: '(R)outine, proactive public health activities have been chronically under-prioritized in terms of investment and stakeholder action, compared with hospital-based health care and disease-specific interventions' (WHO:2022;1). The recent experience of the COVID pandemic makes the case for greater public health investment in the future even stronger.

The third challenge concerns the impact of advances in biomedical genomic research over the course of the last three decades. The completion of the thirteen-year long Human Genome Project (HGP) in 2003 opened up the potential for the development individualised molecular-based clinical diagnostics and treatment. These developments appeared to represent the possibility for what has subsequently become known as 'personalised' or 'precision' medicine being made available to all. Yet the translation of genomic research into routine clinical practice within health systems has been slow and faces substantial challenges. One of the main factors to be considered is the role played by the large pharmaceutical corporations ('Big Pharma') in this process. Not only in its reluctance to invest in the research and development of new drugs to meet emerging health needs, in particular new vaccines and pharmacogenomic interventions, whilst also seeking to maximise their profitability at the expense of national health systems that can ill afford any increase in spending. This is an area of governmental concern that can be broadly categorised under the heading 'pharmaceutical policy'; the focus of this final chapter of this section of the book.

Note

1 There is an important distinction that should be drawn between the concept of health inequality and that of health inequity which are linked but not interchangeable concepts. Social inequities (discussed in many of the chapters in this book) relates to the unequal distribution

of resources between different population groups that result in different levels of access to services – one example would be access to health services based on income in predominantly market-based health care systems, i.e. the USA. Social inequalities in health outcome reflect fundamental social divisions reflecting differences in material wealth, social class, gender, and ethnicity that have long-term implications for the health and life chances of individuals.

Reference
World Health Organisation (2022) *Essential Public Health Functions: a sustainable approach to ensure multi-sectoral actions for population health.* www.who.int (accessed 02/24).

CHAPTER 8

The challenge of integrating health and long-term social care provision

The demographic shift

The overwhelming majority of high-income countries (HICs) have experienced a significant demographic change over the past few decades, that is the trend towards increasingly ageing populations. It part this reflects the overall increase in life expectancy in HICs, but this demographic shift has also occurred in combination with historically low fertility rates below the minimum population replacement requirement. Additionally, there is the more uncertain factor of increasing levels of inward migration. Together these demographic developments are often portrayed as resulting in an ever-increasing social 'burden' of 'dependent' older people. The challenge for policy is to be able to effectively address the increasing need for effective social and long-term care support for our ageing populations, but for too long this challenge has been eschewed by governments in HIC's. The failure to build resilience into our systems of health and social care means that today these services are in grave danger of complete collapse.

To view population ageing as a 'burden' is just one cultural-political perspective, but it is one that has had a disproportional impact in framing the debate about how to address the funding of health and social care services. It is not by chance that one of the key analytical concepts that is drawn upon focuses on the implications for the economy rather less than the social and personal implication of long-term disability and illness that are associated with older age. This concept is known as the 'old age dependency-ratio' (OADR) and it measures the percentage of people aged 65 and over, for every 100 people of working age. With the decline in the average family size in the majority of HICs, the numbers moving into adulthood and employment as a proportion of the total population are gradually being reduced. Figure 8.1 shows the projections for the OADR in five selected HICs plus India and China, up to 2075 (OECD:2023). The upward trend is consistent for all countries, including India and China (although the latter two are currently at a much lower base OADR level.

In the European Union, the combined population of the member states is set to shrink by 5% between 2019 (447 million – current) and 2070 (424 million – projected), while the working-age population (20–64) will decrease by 15.5% over this same period, falling from 265 million in 2019 to 217 million in 2070. Therefore the average OADR across the EU member states is projected to sharply increase over the long term, with the equivalent of less than two working-age persons for every person aged 65 and over by 2070. This EU projection is said to take account of the average rate of fertility, life expectancy as well as migration flow dynamics (EC:2021;4). The predicted demographic change in

DOI: 10.4324/9781003564249-12

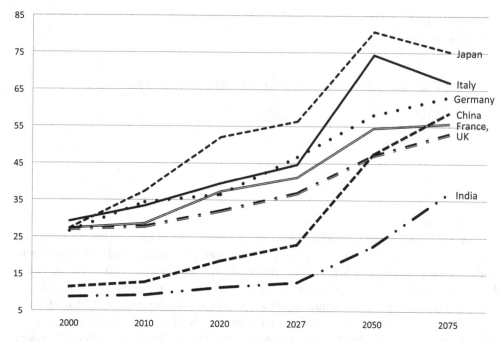

Figure 8.1 Old-Age dependency-ratio by total percentage projections for selected countries 2000–75 (Adapted from OECD (2023)).

the UK is somewhat different, in that the Office of National Statistics has projected a population *increase* of 14.2% in the period 2021–2046, but thereafter the curve flattens until 2075 (ONS:2024). This difference between these projections is that the ONS assumes that there will be a higher rate of long-term net migration (up until 2035) into the UK than within the EU member states. While the absolute numbers of older people are projected to increase significantly in the UK over the next thirty years, if the projected migratory numbers prove correct, then this will result in a smaller increase in the percentage OADR as migrants are typically of working age.

These projected OADRs, in combination with other social and economic developments, clearly set out the challenge for policy-makers of how to balance the requirements of the economy and the robustness of public finances as the working (and therefore income tax-paying) population reduces in proportion to the rising numbers of pension claimants, and the increasing need for health and long-term care (LTC)[1] services.

Ageing societies and determinants of health care spending

Older people do not constitute a homogenous group in society. Retirement from employment does not necessarily mean a significant reduction in income. On the contrary, for those who formally were employed in well-remunerated jobs with occupational pensions attached, and who now own their homes outright with no mortgage to pay, retirement offers many opportunities for continuing health and leisure. When care support does become necessary as morbidities and disabilities accumulate in older age, then people with high incomes and wealth are likely to have sufficient personal savings to ensure that the cost of paying for professional care in their own home or in a residential home is less of a concern. But for those who have spent a lifetime in low-paid jobs with no occupational pension, and without the opportunity to save or purchase their own home, the experience of retirement can be daunting. A significant reduction in income post-retirement may only exacerbate what is likely to be a poorer health status given the known inequalities in health outcome that exist between social classes.

The European Commission has published an 'Ageing Report' every third year since 2003, with the 7th iteration published in 2021[2] (EC:2021) The Ageing Report presents an assessment of the social and economic impact of ageing populations on health and LTC spending in EU member states, projected over a 50-year time period. The 2021 Report projects an increase in older age-related expenditure of an average 2% above current GDP spending in member states, but with some member countries projected as seeing rises as high as 4–6% above their current GDP spend (EC:2021;8). In response, many member states have already begun to instigate reforms to their pension entitlement arrangements in order to ensure the long-term fiscal sustainability of these schemes. These reforms typically include reductions in the benefit-to-contribution ratio, as well as changes to the statutory age of retirement, with the aim of reducing the share of GDP spent on state pensions in the future. Reforms to current inadequate systems of long-term care have been less forthcoming as will be discussed below.

Age-related profiles of health care expenditure in EU member states show that, perhaps unsurprisingly, spending per capita (as % of GDP) increases for men after the age of 55, and for women after the age of 60, reflective of the former's higher morbidity rates in older age. Increases in life expectancy combined with a rising proportion of the elderly in the population, 'leads to increased demand for services over a longer period of the lifetime, increasing total lifetime health care expenditure' (EC:2021;107). However, it is also salient to bear in mind that the trend in rising health care expenditure is not a recent phenomenon.[3] In the 1960s and 1970s, the rise reflected increasing demand for health care services as populations increased in size within HICs, primarily in response to improvements in the standard of living. Today, the demographic shift is of a different order. It is not the population as a whole that is increasing, rather it is the proportion of elderly within that population.

Forty years ago, as the demographic shift towards longevity became clear, there was an initial optimism which reflected the notion of 'healthy older ageing' that was underpinned by what became known as the *compression of morbidity* hypothesis. This epidemiological concept assumed that disability and ill-health would become compressed towards the later period of life at a faster pace than the rise in mortality. People were expected to not only live longer but also in better health for longer. This thesis was fuelled in part by an optimism surrounding the continued rise in living standards, but ultimately shown to be false because of the collateral consequences of economic globalisation, climate change, and a failure to systematically address social inequalities. The initial optimism that health costs could be held in check as populations aged also reflected the initial promise of new digital medical technologies, the assumption being that innovation would reduce costs as diagnostics and medicines improved. In reality, innovations in medical technology have been variously estimated as contributing somewhere between 25% and 75% of the increase in health expenditure seen over the last 30 years (EC:2021;109).

Nevertheless, the demographic gains in life expectancy and reduction in mortality rates have not in practice resulted in equivalent gains in disability-free life expectancy. Many of the extra years of life are today marked by the debilitating experience of physical dependency, multi-morbidity, and social isolation, a process that became known as the *expansion of morbidity*. Medical technology alone can do little to reduce morbidity rates and maintain good health status for longer into older age, It has become an epidemiological given that the primary determinants that influence health status over a lifetime are social, economic, and environmental, and this was also the default assumption of the compression of morbidity thesis discussed above. On this basis, rising health care expenditure must be assessed alongside the proportion of public expenditure directed to limiting the lifetime impact of social and economic factors on health status, beyond the provision of health care in and of itself.

A further determinant of the rising health care expenditure is the costs of 'human capital'. Health care professionals are an essential component of health service provision and the care sector is much more labour-intensive than other employment sectors within the economy. It is on this basis that any changes associated with workforce costs and productivity will have a direct impact on both provision and health care expenditure. This can include improvements to the heath professional-patient ratio in order to raise the quality of care, as well as increases in remuneration to order to retain expensively trained, skilled, and highly qualified staff.

Finally, there are potentially foreseeable but unpredictable factors ('known unknowns') that could contribute to significant but time-restricted rises in health care spending. The clearest example would be infectious disease outbreaks that lead to national epidemics and even pandemics. The human cost and the resource implications of the COVID-19 pandemic in 2020 through to 2022 will continue to be felt for many years, despite the rapid development of effective mRNA vaccination programmes. In recent years, we have witnessed the Ebola virus disease epidemic in West Africa (2013–16), as well as the Zika virus disease epidemic in a variety of geographical regions across the world in 2015. Epidemics spread across national borders, they are difficult to anticipate and result in dramatic increases in the rates of morbidity and mortality. In medium- (MICs) and low-income countries (LICs), as more people move to live and work in urban areas, and as their populations grow, and with the additional factor of the impact of climate change, inevitably new transmissible variants of viruses will emerge to set further challenges for health systems across the globe.

Ageing societies and fiscal policy: future scenarios

The European Commission Ageing Report (EC:2021) has set out a range of projected scenarios for health care spending resulting from the increase in older people as a proportion of population in member states, from the present day up until 2075. The report sets out 12 such scenarios, but for conciseness given that there is quite a lot of overlap between these scenarios, just four are outlined below.

(i) The *demographic scenario* attempts to isolate the 'pure' effects of ageing on health spending and so operates on the assumption that age-specific morbidity rates do not change over time. This scenario is predicated on the 'expansion of morbidity' thesis (see above), where all gains in life expectancy are spent in poorer health. On this basis, current age-related health care spending per capita deemed to be a proxy measure for projected health status,[4] remains stable in real terms over the time period projected. The scenario further assumes that health care costs, and therefore expenditure per capita, evolve in line with GDP per capita. 'This implies that without a change in the age structure of the population and in life expectancy, the share of health care spending in GDP would remain constant over the projection period' (EC:2021;115). On the basis of the 'demographic scenario', the EC Ageing Report predicts an increase in public expenditure on health care (but <u>not</u> THE) averaging 1.2% of GDP across EU member states over the projected period (EC:2021;123).

(ii) The *healthy ageing scenario* is rather more optimistic about future health spending as it is predicated on the 'compression of morbidity' thesis. This scenario envisages a fall in rates of morbidity in older age alongside a decline in the mortality rate. This scenario results in a much smaller projected increase in health spending per capita GDP for most EU member countries. On the basis of this scenario, the EC Ageing Report predicts an increase in public expenditure on health care averaging just 0.3% of GDP across EU member states over the projected period (EC:2021;124).

(iii) The *labour intensity scenario* assumes that the unit costs of health care spending are driven by changes in the productivity of the labour force, rather than growth in the national income. This assumption follows from the fact that health and social care provision is a highly labour-intensive sector (see above). So contrary to the demographic scenario, in this particular scenario 'the cost of public provision of health care is supply- rather than demand-driven' (EC:2021;116). Health spending costs are therefore assumed to grow in line with wages, linked to increases in productivity. As productivity rates generally rise at a faster rate than GDP per capita, so the unit costs of health care are driven by these wage increases. In this scenario the EC Ageing Report predicts an increase in public expenditure averaging 0.5% of GDP *additional* to the demographic scenario projection, across EU member states (EC:2021;127).

(iv) The *non-demographic determinants scenario* looks to estimate the influence of determinants other than demographics on health care spending. It therefore includes national income, new technology and other institutional factors in the calculation. It also assesses the extent to which health care that is currently funded through SHI and/or PHI contributions can accommodate to the challenge of a reduction in net contributions as the proportion of those in paid employment decreases. It is on this basis that this scenario is also termed the 'excess cost growth' model. The scenario seeks to challenge the (false) assumption, implicit in a number of other possible scenarios, 'that past trends of health care expenditure related to these drivers will disappear in the future' (EC:2021;118). On the basis of this 'non-demographic determinants scenario', the EC Ageing Report predicts an increase in public expenditure on health care averaging a much more significant rise of 3.1% of GDP across EU member states over the projected period (EC:2021;127).

In the context of these projected health care spending scenarios, it should also be noted that the OADR is currently calculated on the basis of the average retirement age being 64 years. However, given that these scenarios are set over a 50-year period, the projected public fiscal deficits in all the scenarios cited must be subject to critique. Many HIC have a legislative timetable already in place to push back the age of eligibility further still over the next twenty years. It is also now increasingly common to find people working beyond the statutory state pension age. This may be out of financial necessity, reflecting the inadequacies of a state pension income, or because relatively good health in older age facilitates extending years in paid employment. The latter outcome would represent a realisation of the 'compression of morbidity' thesis, but it is also quite possible to be in employment (the Office of National Statistics in the UK use the rather confusing terminology of being 'economically active') with increasing disability if employers are able to provide the appropriate support. One associated factor that has already been discussed is the impact of the rise in migrant populations in Europe who have a much younger than average age profile, and so can add to the numbers of net contributors in the OADR.

Long-term care provision

Austria hosted the first United Nations World Assembly on Ageing in 1982, from which emerged the 'Vienna International Plan of Action on Ageing'. The primary goals of this Plan of Action were, 'to strengthen the capacities of countries to deal effectively with the ageing of their populations and with the special concerns and needs of their elderly' (UN:1982). These underpinning goals were later to be adopted by the UN General Assembly in its 'Principles for Older People' (UN:1991). These principles sought to 'add life to the years that have been added to life' through the promotion of independence, participation, care, self-fulfilment, and dignity of older citizens and remain 'the foundation for developing national legislation of ageing and older persons around the world' (Leichsenring & Sidorenko:2024;4). These long-established UN principles can serve as the gauge by which we might assess the adequacy of contemporary national provision of LTC services for older people, and on this basis many countries do not measure up.

LTC provision is intended to meet the 'needs'[5] of people living with reduced functional capacity linked to either physical or cognitive limitations. The most effective form of LTC provision is predicated on the principle that providing early support enables individuals to meet the requirements of 'activities of daily living'[6] (ADLs). Early intervention means that individuals are enabled to maintain their personal independence for as long as possible and within their own home. However, if an individual's level of physical or cognitive disability has developed to the point where providing support at home becomes unfeasible, then it may become necessary to support them in a professionally staffed residential setting. In virtually all European systems, LTC provision is primarily delivered within an individual's own home. In the UK, this home-based support is more usually termed 'social care', but the nomenclature of support does vary from country to country.

At this point it is important to take time-out from describing the structures of LTC provision to emphasis that fact that the primary providers of support across Europe for those with a reduced capacity for independent living are not the formal systems, but rather the life partners and family members of these individuals who are generally referred to as 'informal carers'. For a long period of time in the UK, little was known about the numbers of people who had voluntarily taken on the role of informal carer.

It was only in 2001 that a series of questions about care arrangements in the home were included in the national census that is carried out once every decade. These questions sought to elicit information about those living with a disability, and the amount of time family members spent providing ADL support. Informal care is provided at very little public cost, but it does come at considerable personal cost for the carers themselves. There can be financial costs if the carer has to reduce their hours of employment or give up full-time paid work altogether in order to provide care. The 'costs' of caring often go beyond the purely financial, it can be physically demanding, and the unremitting demands of providing care to a loved one can also be psychologically stressful, and can contribute to poorer health outcomes for the informal carers themselves. The majority of European countries have chosen to separate the provision of health care services from that of LTC services, and the universal right to comprehensive health care does not generally extend to a universal entitlement to LTC free at the point of need.

In the UK, it is estimated that 24% of men and 28% of women aged 65 and over are living with at least one ADL deficit that requires support, rising to 52% for those aged over 80 years. Those requiring support who are living with two or more ADL deficits equate to 15% of all adults aged 65–69, and 40% of those aged 80 and over in the UK (ONS:2023). Yet examined in terms of public expenditure (measured as spending per LTC recipients as a percentage of GDP per capita), across all EU member states, spending on LTC does not match the increases there have been in age-related health care expenditure. Estimating LTC costs per recipient is a more complex equation than at first might be assumed. Significant numbers of those requiring care are younger disabled individuals who require support for a life time. The settings in which care is provided is also a major factor in expenditure, for example the provision of care as against institutional care reflects the degree of disability not age per se (EC:2021;139).

A mix of public and private funded LTC provision can be found across the EU member states and the UK, but the one constant is the essentially fragmentary nature of provision. State or public funding of LTC provision has historically been given a low-policy priority, with the responsibility for provision distributed across government departments (EC:2021;138). Nonetheless, in belated recognition of the fact that ageing populations will require more investment in care support services, 'many countries have started to reform their LTC systems, e.g. by changing eligibility criteria or altering the financing of LTC. These measures altered the scope and functioning of many established LTC systems. As a consequence, it has become increasingly difficult to describe and categorize existing LTC systems' (Ariaans et al:2021;609). These authors have gone on to develop an updated comparative typology of LTC provision[7] to be found across 25 OECD member countries. This exercise draws on the methodology of cluster analysis in order to bracket national systems together predicated on four assessment dimensions each with their own set of quantitative and qualitative indicators: (i) supply, (ii) public-private mix, (iii) access regulation, and (iv) performance. Utilising this cluster method, the comparative analysis identified six ideal-typologies, these are outlined below. It should be noted that the terms 'low', 'medium', and 'high' that appear in the ideal-type clusters below are utilised as an indicator of the average overall functionality of these types of LTC systems found in 25 OECD member states (Ariaans et al:2021;612–614).

(a) *The residual public system*: Former Soviet bloc countries with low levels of supply (overall expenditure, numbers of beds and recipients of care in institutions), but with no access restrictions or means-testing.

(b) *The private supply system*: Germany and Finland, which have medium levels of supply but one of the lowest shares of public expenditure. No restrictions on cash benefits, and access to the system is not means tested.

(c) *The public supply system*: Mainly Nordic countries with high levels of supply and the highest levels of proportional expenditure among OECD member countries. No means-testing, and the system benefits are in kind (good and services rather than monetary benefits). Performance measured in life expectancy and health status is low.

(d) *The evolving public supply system*: Japan and South Korea are cited as examples. Access to the system is granted without means-testing, but medium to high choice restrictions apply.

(e) *The needs based supply system*: This includes the following member countries, Australia, Belgium, Switzerland, Luxembourg, the Netherlands, Slovakia, and Slovenia. Public expenditure is about average but supply is high. In contrast to the private supply type, access is restricted by a high level of means-testing, with above average performance.

(f) *The evolving private needs based supply system*: This includes the UK, France, Spain, New Zealand and the USA, and shares many characteristics of the 'need based supply system', but with the public-private mix tending towards private financing of needs. Access is restricted through means-testing and a low supply of service and low expenditure. Therefore, there is a limited choice of provision, especially in relation to residential care.

Ariaans et al (2021) typology provides the analytical context for a more detailed comparative case study assessment of the strengths and limitations of the Austrian[8] and the English LTC systems as set out below.

Case study 1: the social care system in England

The system of long-term social care in the UK was established in 1990 and is a decentralised model. Local authorities in England, Wales, and Scotland have statutory 'Adult Social Services Responsibilities' that require them to provide social care services in the geographical locality. While in Northern Ireland, it is the health and social care trusts that have this responsibility, the care system being an integrated one in this region (HoC:2014). Funding for social care provision comes from two main sources. Central grants from government (the Scottish and Welsh Assemblies receive a block grant intended to support the statutory responsibilities of these devolved administration's) and local revenue-raising mechanisms. In the year 2023/24, 51% of social care provision revenue expenditure came from Government grants, 31% from local authority raised 'council tax', and 15% from retained local business rates.

UK Government grants to local authorities were cut by 40% in real terms over the decade from 2009/10 to 2019/20, despite the increasing demand for social care services (Atkins & Hoddinott:2020). Post-COVID-19, this underfunding has continued. In 2022/23, although total expenditure on adult social care rose in England rose to £28 billion, this actually represented a 1% cut in real terms compared to 2020/21 (Kings Fund:2024). In 2022–23, there were some 2 million new requests for LTC support additional to those already in support, 600k were from people below the age of 64, and 1.4 million from those aged 65 years of age and over. Nevertheless, despite this rise in requests, the actual number of people age 65 and older who received LTC support either in a residential setting or in their own home was just 550K, a number that has remained more or less static since 2015–16 (NHS Digital:2024).

The long-term social care system operates on a different funding basis than the health care system within England. The National Health Service (NHS) is funded on the principle of 'cost-risk pooling', where the adult population contributes to the total costs of the health system through direct taxation, and services are provided free at the point of need. In relation to the LTC system, while local authorities in England have a statutory duty to provide social care services, anyone who requests publically funded support must undergo an individual means test. If an individual has personal savings of more than £23,250 (*unchanged as of October 2024*) they must then pay for the cost of their care on a sliding scale based on their financial assets. Individuals aged 65 and over, and living in the most deprived areas in England, were twice as likely to need help with their ADLs as adults living in least deprived areas (ONS:2023).Central government grants have never met the resource requirements of English local authorities that would enable them to begin to close the gap between the support needs of those with long-term disabilities and their available levels of social care provision. Yet there is good evidence that functional decline can be halted and even reversed if support is provided at an early stage (Kingston:2017). When interventions arrive only at the point of advanced physical or cognitive chronicity, then this ultimately requires a far greater demand on institutional resources, not to mention the impact on the self-esteem and confidence of the individual concerned. Means-tested systems of provision always result in unmet needs.

Since the post-2009 'austerity budgets', central government grants to local authorities decreased year on year in real terms. This historic underfunding of social care services in England has required local authorities to focus their efforts on what has become known as 'firefighting', managing problems as they arise rather than developing long-term strategies of prevention. This is the basis on which eligibility criteria, tied to an assessment of individual social care needs, were introduced into the system. The imposition of extremely tight eligibility criteria is a crude attempt to manage the demand for LTC that has long outpaced levels of available provision. This has meant that individuals with low- to medium-level physical or cognitive dependency are unlikely to qualify for any support at all. Even prior to the COVID-19 pandemic it was estimated that to meet the expected growth in demand for social care services, and to return spending (relative to demand) to the peak levels seen before austerity, social care would need an additional £10.0bn per year (The Health Foundation:2020).

In March 2024, the House of Commons Committee of Public Accounts produced its 'Report on the state of Adult Social Care in England' (HoC:2024). House of Commons select committees consist of between 10 and 50 elected members of Parliament drawn from across all major political parties. They are charged with considering the outcomes of national policies, scrutinising specific areas of government work and expenditure, and examining proposals for legislation, they also consider evidence taken from expert witness as well as formal submissions. The basis for the investigation of adult social care policy in 2024 (the Public Accounts Committee had reported on social care on many occasions in the past) was the significant delay in the then Conservative government coming forward with detailed policy proposals and a timescale for reforming the system. The government had set out their 'ten-year vision' for fundamental change more than two years previously in 2021 in a White Paper entitled *People at the heart of care*, but no action had been undertaken since that time.

The Committee Report began by questioning whether the introduction of a new structural layer within NHS England, known as Integrated Care Systems (ICS)[9], that followed the 2022 *Health and Care Act,* had made any 'demonstrable difference' to the delivery of social care in England: 'We remain concerned about under-representation of adult social care in health-dominated systems and are deeply sceptical about the feasibility of integrating health and social care when they are funded so differently' (HoC:2024;5). The Report went on to express further concern that the government was not being proactive but simply reacting to on-going crises, when it periodically allocated additional pots of funding to local authorities to deliver care services without any clear mechanism for establishing whether this money was resulting in 'tangible improvements' to the system: 'Patchwork funding and short-term announcements hinder the sector's ability to plan for the long-term and risks undermining delivery of the Department's (of Health and Social care) 10 year vision for adult social care' (HoC:2024;6). Finally, the Report acknowledged the concern of the local authorities in England that they had only been given limited representation on the new Integrated Care Boards (ICBs). While the 2022 *Health and Care Act* now mandated joint decision-making for social care provision between representatives of a local authority and local NHS trusts via the ICBs; 'it is not guaranteed that monies distributed by these means will always be allocated to social care … (the risk was) that it might be absorbed into spending to meet acute health care pressures' (HoC:2024;10). In July 2024, a Labour Government was elected to power. One of their pre-election manifesto commitments was to reform the social care system. The first budget of the new government in October 2024 was an opportunity to demonstrate this commitment through a significant increase in resources. While the NHS received an additional £22bn, local councils in England received just an additional £600m to cover both adult and child social care services. This early opportunity for reform was eschewed. In short, the limitations of the social care system in England have been discussed and debated for decades, but the limited attempts to integrate health and social care structures have failed on the consistent grounds of underinvestment and a lack of political commitment to reform.

Case study 2: the long-term care system in Austria

Austria has some 1.5 million people aged over 65 years, equating to 18% of the total population. A significant proportion of these older Austrians live in rural alpine areas, this presents its own very specific challenges for the delivery of care provision.

A comprehensive LTC system with cash-for-care allowances was established in in 1993, replacing the previous fragmentary arrangements. Funding for these care allowances comes from the Federal Republic government and derived from general taxation, while the decentralised federal state governments are responsible for delivering services in kind. The cash-for-care allowances are not means-tested and are based solely on the outcome of an individual LTC needs assessment. However, the standards and availability of services and facilities, as well as the use of eligibility criteria, do vary considerably across the nine federal states of Austria (Leichsenring et al:2021;34). Some 47,000 professionals provide support for around 70,000 people in LTC residential homes, while a further 18,000 professionals provide home-based care to 153,000 clients. In total, 462K Austrians of all ages were assessed as in need of care in 2018 and on that basis were eligible for federal cash-for-care allowances (BMASGK:2019 – cited in Leichsenring et al:2021;34).

The Austrian LTC system has one notable feature that has been developed over the past 30 years, this is the so-called '24 hour care' model. This provides for the supplementation of family or informal care by live-in self-employed personal carers. These carers are mainly drawn from neighbouring Eastern European Countries and are attracted by the significant wage differentials for equivalent work in their own country. While paid live-in care can be found in other national LTC systems, including England, the Austrian model of live-in personal care is closely regulated. Since 2007 it has been according a special status within the Austrian LTC system, with dedicated funding and regulated conditions of employment for these 'personal carers'. In 2018, 7% of older people assessed as in need of LTC received '24-hour care' in their own homes, equating to some 66,000 personal carers for 33,000 older citizens. Yet the personal carer system is also seen having resulted in a 'dualisation' of the LTC workforce, dividing it in terms of migratory status, as well as skills, remuneration and precarious working conditions: 'It thus competes with and likely hampers the development of integrated care and community-based care services' (Leichsenring et al:2021;34).

In the case of both the Austrian and English 'private needs based supply', see Ariaans et el (2021) type 'f' above, provision of care support is predicated on the construction of older persons as 'consumers'. It also built around the assumption that private provider competition enables individuals to choose from among a variety of types of care services that meet their individual care needs. But this type of LTC consumerism brings with it the risk of individuals making uninformed decisions when objective information about the suitability of these care services is often scarce (Eggers et al:2022;415). Predominantly private market LTC systems have been associated with low quality of care and poor working conditions for staff. Care workers in the private sector frequently experience low pay and high job insecurity, the resulting poor morale amongst staff does not generally engender the delivery of high-quality care provision.

The impact of the COVID-19 pandemic in both Austria and England clearly demonstrated the weaknesses and deficiencies of both LTC systems. While Austria experienced a lower incidence of the disease and subsequent COVID-related mortality during the first wave of the pandemic, the 'collateral effects' of focusing on the response of the acute secondary care system to the exclusion of residential LTC, in particular, served to exacerbate the long-term impact of the virus (Leichsenring et al:2021;36). These 'collateral effects' were also very much a feature of the management of the pandemic in care homes in England. During the first wave of the pandemic in 2020, 23.9% (75,664) of the deaths of care home residents involved COVID-19 (ONS:2022). This is a considerably higher proportion of deaths from COVID-19 than occurred in the elderly population as a whole. At the high point of the pandemic, the notable lack of coordination and integration of care across both the Austrian and English LTC systems was devastating for older members of the population living with multimorbities and at greater health risk.

Conclusion: meeting the challenge of integrating long-term health and social care services

Meeting the societal challenge of constructing a health and social care system to effectively meet the rising demand for LTC care support requires a more expansive vision than the one-dimensional perspective found in many countries that focuses solely on the setting of pre-determined cost-efficiency targets. Any fundamental improvement in provision can only be achieved if the first crucial step towards integrating the structures of health care and long-term social care provision is undertaken to create a balanced and responsive universal care system. Integration also means addressing the inequities found across health and social care provision, where the majority of resources continue go to the acute secondary care hospital sector to the detriment of the preventative, primary care and LTC sectors.

Integrating long-term health care services is not some radical alternative to the dual systems of care that are currently in place across the majority of European countries. The experience of the COVID-19 pandemic was a reality-check that clearly demonstrated the consequences of an over-reliance on the private market for care provision. Many governments have subsequently began to reassess their LTC policies. In England, the *Health and Care Act* of 2022 which sought to promote greater integration of services is discussed above, but the European Commission has also more recently rolled out what it calls its 'Integrated Care Flagship Technical Support Project'. Its goal is to provide 'tailored work packages' that provide support to ministries of health and the ministries of social affairs within its Member states, to enable them to: '(D)esign and implement structural reforms in the areas of health, social care and long-term care (in order to) strengthen the coordination between these sectors and the integration of the different levels of care provision, by putting the person at the centre of services' (EC:2022).

Yet achieving integration of provision is not simply a matter of national governments issuing top-down edicts that urge closer cooperation between the health care and LTC sectors.[10] It is also necessary to develop new integrated structures that can pool financing across all care (health and social care) services, this is a particular challenge for those systems that that are reliant on social health insurance (SHI) funding, less so for those receiving the bulk of funding through direct taxation. An integrated system is also one that effectively manages the professional care workforce. The challenge here is to overcome the imbalance in power and influence that continues to exist between the acute medical sector and local authority providers of care support services. Integrating care services requires a restructuring of the mechanisms of organisational governance, and places the needs of the patient and the citizen at its centre.

Notes

1 In this chapter, the term 'long term care' (LTC) will be utilised to cover, following the WHO definition, 'a broad range of personal, social and medical services and support that ensure people with, or at risk of, a significant loss of intrinsic capacity (due to mental, or physical illness or disability) can maintain a level of functional ability consistent with their basic rights and human dignity' (WHO:2022). In the UK, the umbrella term 'social care' covers essentially the same range of provision.

2 The 8th Edition of the Ageing Report was scheduled to be published by the European Commission in Spring 2024, unfortunately this was after the final manuscript for this textbook had been completed.

3 See Figure 4.3 and its linked discussion in Chapter 4.

4 Age-profiled health care expenditure is not per se, a measure of health status, but the report utilises this as its proxy measure ... 'given the lack of a reliable and comparable data, it is plausible to assume that the shape of the profiles follows the evolution of health status over the lifespan' (EC:2021;115).

5 The notion of 'needs' in a health and social context is a contested one. Bradshaw's (1972) taxonomy of needs is frequently cited in the social policy literature as the definitive starting point for any conceptualisation of social need. It has also been utilised to critique the flawed assumption that most people's social needs are met by the welfare state because health and social care services are universal, that is, available to everybody in society according to their need. The taxonomy is built upon the premise that needs are *socially constructed,* by which it is meant that human social needs are not universal and transcendental, but are a product of a particular society at a particular historical moment. The taxonomy developed by Bradshaw identified four possible ways of defining individual needs, set out in a hierarchical form as follows: (1) *Felt Need:* when people are conscious of needs but are not explicitly recognised and remains hidden. (2) *Expressed Needs:* When needs are known about and become demands. (3) *Normative Needs:* Defined according to professional norms or standards. (4) *Comparative Needs:* Introduces the notion of social justice. Is one social group getting something others are not?

6 ADLs are defined as activities related to personal care and mobility about the home that are fundamental to independent daily living.

7 The Ariaans et al (2021) typology is just one of several such typologies that can be found within the social/health policy literature. An even more ambitious typology of global LTC systems that was published in the same year can be found in Rothgang et al (2021). The latter typology adopts an 'actor-centred approach' to deriving distinct LTC typologies.

8 Although Austria is a (founding) member of the OECD, it was excluded from Ariaans et al (2021) analysis because of 'data limitations'. However, based on previous studies, these same authors included Austria in their 'private supply' typology cluster, together with Germany and Finland.

9 Discussed in detail in relation to the NHS in Chapter 7.

10 See Figure 7.2 in Chapter 7.

References

Ariaans, M, Linden, P and Wendt, C (2021) Worlds of long-term care: a typology of OECD countries, *Health Policy*, vol. 125, 609–617.

Atkins, G and Hoddinott, S (2020) *Local Government Funding in England – Briefing 10th March 2020.* http://www.instituteforgovernment.org.uk (accessed 10/23).

BMASGK – Bundesministerium für Arbeit, Soziales, Gesundheit und Konsumentenschutz (2019) *Österreichischer Pflegevorsorgebericht 2018.* Vienna. BMASGK.

Bradshaw, J (1972) 'Taxonomy of social need' in McLachlan, G (ed) *Problems and Progress in Medical Care; Essays on Current Research.* Oxford. Oxford University Press, pp 71–82.

Eggers, T, Grages, C and Pfau-Effinger, B (2022) How culture influences the strengthening of market principles in conservative welfare states: the case of long-term care policy, *International Journal of Social Welfare*, vol. 33, no. 413–426.

European Commission (2021) *2021 Ageing report: Institutional Paper 138.* Luxembourg. EC.

European Commission (2022) *Flagship Technical Support Project – Towards person-centred integrated care*. https://reform-support.ec.europa.eu (accessed 02/24).

Health and Care Act (2022) https://legislation.gov.uk/ukpga/2022/31/contents (accessed 01/2023).

Health Foundation (2020) *The Social Care Funding Gap*. www.health.org.uk (accessed 12/2022).

House of Commons (2014) *Local Authorities Public Health Responsibilities (England) Standard Note – SN06844*. London. House of Commons Library.

House of Commons Committee of Public Accounts (2024) *Reforming Adult Social Care in England: 22nd Report of Session 2023–24*. London. House of Commons Library.

Kings Fund (2024) *Social Care 360: Expenditure*. www.kingsfund.org.uk (accessed 03/2024).

Kingston, A et al (2017) Is late-life dependency increasing or not? A comparison of the cognitive function and ageing studies (CFAS), *Lancet*, vol. 390, 1676–1684.

Leichsenring, K, Schmidt, A and Staflinger, H (2021) Fractures in the Austrian model of long-term care: what are the lessons from the first wave of the COVID-19 pandemic? *Journal of Long-Term Care*, Feb 2nd, 33–42.

Leichsenring, K and Sidorenko, A (2024) 'Introduction: why do we need a research agenda for ageing and social policy in the 21st century?' in Leichsenring, K and Sidorenko, A (eds) *A Research Agenda for Ageing and Social Policy*. Cheltenham. Edward Elgar Publishing, pp 3–18

NHS Digital (2024) *Adult Social Care Statistics in England: An Overview*. https://digital.nhs.uk (accessed 03/2024).

OECD (2023) *Pensions at a Glance 2023: OECD and G20 Indicators*. https://doi.org/10.1787?678055dd-en (accessed 02/2024).

Office of National Statistics (2022). *Deaths involving COVID-19 in the care sector, England and Wales: Deaths registered between week ending 20th March 2020 and week ending 21st January 2022*. www.ons.gov.uk (accessed 02/2024).

Office of National Statistics (2023) *Health Survey for England, 2021, part 2*. www.digital.nhs.uk (accessed 03/2024).

Office of National Statistics (2024) *National Population projections: 2021-based interim*. www.ons.gov.uk (accessed 02/2024).

Rothgang, H, Fischer, J, Sternkopf, M and Doetter, L (2021) *The classification of distinct long-term care systems worldwide: the empirical application of an actor-centred multi-dimensional typology*. Bremen, Germany. SOCIUM Working Papers 12.

United Nations (1982) *Report of the World Assembly on Ageing, Vienna 26 July to 6 August 1982: A/CONF.113/31*. https://www.un.org/ (accessed 03/2024).

United Nations (1991) *General Assembly – Forty-Sixth Session – Implementation of the International Plan of Action on Ageing 46/91*. https://documents.un.org/doc/resolution/gen/nr0/581/79/img/nr058179 (accessed 03/2024).

World Health Organisation (2022) *Questions and answers/Long-term care*. www.who.int (accessed 01/24).

CHAPTER 9

The challenge of widening the scope of public health policy

An ideal-type public health system?

The Faculty of Public Health (FPH) is a membership association for over 4,000 public health professionals in the UK and across the world; it also acts as a standard setting institution for the training, and examining of specialist public health practice. In a recent publication entitled 'Functions and standards of a Public Health System' (FPH:2020), the Faculty set out what it regards as the three essential 'domains' of public health practice. These domains align strongly with the WHO 'Essential Public Health Operations' strategy (WHO:2022).

The first of these domains is termed *Health Protection*. Here the focus is on environmental health hazards, the need to improve the quality of the air we breathe, the water we drink, and the food we eat, and effective upstream infectious disease prevention and control. Public health interventions in this domain involve collaborative activities that necessarily go beyond the conventional bounds of biomedically orientated health systems, and include not only the statutory local authorities, health and safety regulatory institutions, but also voluntary groups and other partner organisations. The second domain is *Health Improvement*. Here the primary focus is on reducing social inequalities in health outcomes and the promotion of health and well-being. Once again, in order to make progress in this domain partnership working across both the formal and informal sectors of public and civil spheres of society is seen as a key requirement.[1] The third domain *Health Services* is a more conventional area for the involvement of public health professionals, but here the FPH argues for a much greater degree of integration of public health services than is currently the case in the UK and beyond. It argues that the wider concerns of population health prevention and the promotion of well-being should be 'mainstreamed' in all areas of health service planning, commissioning, and development. The conjecture being that integrating social and health care services and engaging local communities in the development of services that meet their needs, is both a more efficient use of resources as well as addressing the concerns around equitable access and social inequalities in health (FPH:2020).

This ideal-type[2] public health system is seen as being able to integrate these three domains of intervention to address the overriding threats to population health. Yet the reality of public health provision in the UK remains far removed from this model. Since the inception of the National Health Service (NHS) over 75 years ago, the level of public health funding has remained low in comparison with the secondary health care sector.

DOI: 10.4324/9781003564249-13

Social inequalities in health and public health policy

The historic role of the state in maintaining the health of the population, or more precisely limiting health risk, has evolved in a responsive series of fits and starts in Britain, rather than in a progressive arc. The early legislative interventions in the nineteenth century were primarily concerned with limiting the spread of infectious disease, through investment in the building of sewers and sanitation facilities, the provision of clean water supplies, and other environmental improvement programmes. Today, a wide range of public health interventions are in place to limit threats to population health that extend from child vaccination programmes, to legislation to reduce road traffic accident deaths and injuries, tobacco advertising bans, water fluoridation to reduce dental caries, sexual health education in schools, as well as support for a host of health promotion activities. But these public health initiatives, with the exception of vaccination programmes, have frequently been under-resourced and small in scope and scale. The UK Government has been reluctant to intervene to address the health outcomes of what are often characterised as individual 'lifestyle choices'. Since the effective ending of the Labour Government 'Programme of Action' to reduce inequalities in health (discussed below) in 2010, there has been a marked unwillingness to develop any systematic cross-government strategy to address the ever-widening gap in social inequalities in health outcome.

In the public health canon, the first disease prevention interventions in Britain begin with Dr John Snow and the Cholera epidemic of 1854. John Snow was a practising doctor who as early as 1849 had published an essay on *The Mode of Communication of Cholera*. This was at a time when research into the mode of disease spread was very much in its early stages, Louis Pasteur in France had yet to publish his microbiological findings, and some thirty years prior to Koch's definitive work on the Germ Theory of Disease. During the 1854 cholera epidemic, Snow, who both lived and practiced in the Soho district of Central London, set about interviewing local residents to see if he could determine the pattern of disease spread. He combined his social survey with a microscopic examination of the local water supplies; the information he then acquired enabled him to identify the source of the epidemic as a public water pump this he famously put out of action by removing its handle, after which the incidence of cholera in this district rapidly declined. This case illustrated the limitations of clinical medicine at this time, but more particularly it led onto a gradual understanding that the origins of infectious disease frequently lay in unsanitary social and environmental conditions. Although the introduction of the Public Health Acts of 1848 and 1874 preceded the establishment of the science of bacteriology by several decade, this legislation did much to ensure that clean water and sewage systems were constructed and maintained leading to significant reduction in the rates of communicable disease mortality, especially amongst young children.

By the early twentieth century, innovations in the science of bacteriology had led onto the first pharmacological treatments for infectious disease and culminated in the discovery of penicillin in 1929, the first antibiotic to be isolated (but not produced in sufficient quantities for public use until 1946). This was also the period when bioscience began to be systematically incorporated into the knowledge-base of medical professional training, reflected in more effective methods of medical treatment and surgery. But by the middle of the twentieth century, the earlier understanding of disease prevention at source had become over-shadowed by the notion of a 'pill for every ill' and medical 'silver bullets'. Following the Second World War, the early assumption of government was that the creation of the NHS would improve health for all and eradicate social inequalities in health outcomes. The provision of a universal health care system free at the point of need did indeed erode many of the pre-existing inequities in health care provision, but on its own clinical medicine could not eliminate inequalities in health that primarily derived from differences in social and material life chances within the population. Although the general standard of health for all improved in the early post-war years, as measured by average levels of life expectancy, differences in health outcome, as measured by the differential rate of mortality between social classes, failed to narrow. While the existence of such inequalities was not denied, the official view in the 1960s was that the primary cause of this persistent gap in health outcomes was individual health behaviour and so not the responsibility of government.

It was not until the late 1970s that the weight of evidence from social epidemiological research was convincing enough for the then Labour government to set-up an official commission to investigate social inequalities in health and to produce a set of recommendations for government to act on. The final report to be known as 'The Black Report' (DHSS:1979), named after Sir Douglas Black, then President of the Royal College of Physicians who chaired the commission, was set for publication in late 1979. The report concluded that risks to health were primarily associated with social disadvantage (as measured by socio-economic class) that clustered together and accumulated over the course of a lifetime. Unequal health outcomes were seen as determined by a complex interaction of health behaviours linked to the social, environmental, and material circumstances in which people lived and worked. It was further concluded that poorer health outcomes were not limited to the minority of the population living below the official poverty line, but should be seen as existing across a social class *gradient* of outcomes. The Report was at the point of publication when the newly elected Conservative government, led by Margaret Thatcher, come into power. The new government not only chose to ignore all the report's carefully considered evidence and recommendations, but it also attempted to limit access to the report's findings by refusing official publication, only agreeing to photocopy some 250 copies that were eventually distributed on a Bank Holiday Monday. However, the findings and the recommendations of the Black Report did eventually become widely known following the publication of a short version produced in paperback by the commercial publisher, Penguin Books and available at an affordable price.

Over the following two decades, a period that saw four successive Conservative governments, social inequalities in health outcome never once became a policy issue for government. When the New Labour government came to power in 1997, it set about acting upon its long-held commitment to addressing health inequalities. It commissioned the Chief Medical Officer, Sir Donald Acheson, to produce an independent inquiry into the current state of inequalities in health along the lines of the Black Report that had been produced two decades earlier. The evidence marshalled in the final report (Acheson:1998) once again, convincingly demonstrated that a widening health gap existed between socio-economic classes in Britain. The preface to the Acheson report stated, 'There is convincing evidence that, provided an appropriate agenda of policies can be defined and given priority, many of these inequalities are remediable'. The report went onto make 39 recommendations, but emphasised the need for government action to be taken across a 'broad front'. The report concluded, in somewhat clunky language, that a broad front preventative approach would reflect '(T)he scientific evidence that health inequalities are the outcome of causal chains which run back into and from the basic structure of society. Such an approach is also necessary because many of the factors are interrelated. It is likely to be less effective to focus solely on one point if complementary action is not in place which influences a linked factor in another policy area. Policies need to be both "upstream" and "downstream"' (Acheson:1998;12).

The Labour government accepted the main recommendations of the report in full which were then incorporated within its own policy programme for public health published the following year and entitled, *Saving Lives: Our Healthier Nation* (DoH:1999). This White Paper committed the government to the setting of national and local targets for the reduction of health inequalities, the first time that health targets had ever been set. Four years later, the Department of Health produced its detailed strategy, entitled *Tackling Health Inequalities: A Programme for Action* (DoH:2003). In developing its strategy, the government was quite explicit that success was to be judged on the basis of whether or not it met the following two targets: (a) 'Starting with children under one year, by 2010 to reduce by at least 10 per cent the gap in mortality between manual groups and the population as a whole'. (b) 'Starting with Health Authorities, to reduce by at least 10% the gap between the quintile of the area with the lowest life expectancy at birth and the population as a whole' (DoH:2003;6). Similar to the recommendations of the 1979 Black Report, this strategy emphasised the importance of working across all levels of government (at local, regional, and national levels) and in partnership with other service providers, as well as with local communities to meet these goals. The integration or 'mainstreaming' of health inequality reduction priorities into the planning and performance outcomes not only of the NHS and local government, but all main government departments of state, was seen as crucial to the success of the strategy.

Over the course of the next seven years, up until its election defeat in 2010, the mainstreaming of social inequalities in health through its strategy of 'joined-up' government was a central theme of New Labour policy. In 2009, the government commissioned the eminent social epidemiologist, Sir Michael Marmot, to lead a review of its *Programme of Action* (DoH:2009). This review concluded that while some progress had been made in meeting the inequalities in health targets in *absolute* terms, there had been no overall reduction in health inequalities in *relative* terms.[3] So while health improvements had occurred across all socio-economic classes against a range of indicators including life expectancy, infant mortality, cardiovascular disease, and cancer, the health gap between disadvantaged groups and the rest of the population had not narrowed. It was on this basis that the review acknowledged: '(T)he drive for health improvement can produce an "inverse care law"[4] effect where the benefits of such programme's accrue to the more advantaged groups who have awareness and knowledge of how to use the system …. (A)n effective response needs to be on a sufficient scale if it is to have an impact' (DoH:2009;para 2, p12). The conclusion of this review was that a reduction of the relative social gap in health outcomes was possible, but could only be achieved by continuing with the effective concerted action strategy across all government departments.

Post-2010, with the election of a Conservative government the strategy of addressing social inequalities in health outcome effectively ended in England and Wales. The implementation of the *Health and Social Care Act* in 2012 brought about a fundamental organisational reform of the NHS.[5] An important element of this legislation was the shifting of the responsibility for determining public health objectives and delivering interventions from national NHS primary care services to the local authorities in England.[6] A new arms-length body, Public Health England, was established with the remit of coordinating and financing public health research and publishing the evidence (noting that this body was re-integrated into the Department of Health in 2021 ostensibly to improve central government response to COVID-19). The ring-fenced funding that had been allocated to NHS primary care services for public health programmes was re-purposed as a central government grant to local authorities. In 2014, when the responsibility for public health programmes was finally transferred, the public health grant that was now shared among all the English and Welsh local authorities was just £3 billion, noting that this was at a time when NHS England was receiving an annual budget of £100 billion. There was a short-lived increase in the value of the public health grant during the COVID-19 pandemic, yet in 2023–24, the central grant stood at just £3.5 billion, this constituted a 13% real terms decrease on a like-for-like basis over the course of a decade (ONS:2023).

The public health grant allocation for 2024–25 represented a below inflation increase at £3.6 billion, plus an additional £300k ring-fenced for drug and alcohol as well as smoking services, was due to be spent on the following range of services and in the following proportions: (i) Drug and Alcohol Services for Adults and Youth (£979k) – 25%. (ii) Children's services including the national child measurement programme (£1.1 billion) – 28%. (iii) Sexual health services (£512k) – 13%. (iv) Obesity prevention for adults and children (£238k) – 6%. (v) Stop smoking (£148k) – 3.8%. (vi) Health protection, public health advice, and health check services (£141k) – 3.6%. (vii) Miscellaneous public health services (£576k) – 15% (The Health Foundation:2024). As is clear from this breakdown, the focus of public health interventions remains one of providing preventive services for individuals and groups with known health risks, there is little financial scope for developing wider initiatives to reduce inequalities in health outcome.

The promise of the Labour government 'Programme of Action' evaporated as soon as the 2008 global financial crises began to hit government revenues. While public money was found to bail out the banks and other major financial institutions, significant cuts occurred in public spending on public health initiatives, and impeded the progress that had already been made in mainstreaming population health risk. Yet research in the field of health economics, primarily using the Quality Adjusted Life Year (QALY) measurement tool,[7] has demonstrated that public health interventions are an effective (and cost-effective) utilisation of public money. Research by Martin et al (2020) has demonstrated that the health gains from public health interventions were 3–4 times that of clinical health care. While a study commissioned by the Health Foundation (2024) has found that each additional year of good health within the population could be achieved through public health programmes at the cost of £3800, compared to £13,500 per year for clinical interventions through the NHS.

The narrow scope of contemporary public health policy

Public health policy in England today is largely set out in broad brush terms by central government, with the responsibility for turning these generalised objectives into practical programmes and activities delegated to underfunded local or regional governments.

Public health programmes in most European countries including the UK rarely have the same level of governance oversight that is expected of the health care services. This situation clearly lends itself to the emergence of a gap between policy intent and the process of implementation, as local factors play out in the interpretation of policy goals.

At one level, as has previously been stated, it should be self-evident that funding public health interventions that include upstream disease prevention programmes and the promotion of healthy environments for all, is the most effective and efficient way to improve the health of populations. Yet it is precisely this potential to go beyond the parameters of what historically has been seen to constitute the remit of a health care system that has led paradoxically, to the marginalisation of public health policy; this is a further example of system 'path-dependency'. in action.[8] As has previously been discussed, the NHS was established primarily as a national hospital-dominated system, with local government authorities given the 'residual' responsibility for public health. The marginalisation of public health activities from the inception of the new health system reflected the institutional authority of senior members of the medical profession and the hegemony of the 'medical model', now consolidated within the decision-making structures of the NHS.[9] The medical model is an essentially reductionist perspective of the 'normal' and the 'pathological' rooted in laboratory research and predicated on the notion of a 'specific aetiology', a linear causal pathway explanation of the causes of ill health. Yet as Pankhurst and Abeysinghe (2016) have noted, 'if this evidence predominantly supports individual-level interventions that have minimal reach and effect across populations, the benefits of being informed by the existing evidence base might be illusory' (p. 667). Non-linear causal explanations of poor health, including for example stressful social and toxic material environments, have generally been excluded from the medical model equation.

A re-organisation of the NHS in 1974 saw public health physicians transferred from local government[10] into the NHS, but their role remained a marginal one marginalised within the mainstream activities of the health service. However, in the early 1980s, following the increasing prominence of social epidemiological research concerned with the causality of social inequalities in health (described above), combined with an increased emphasis on 'health promotion' in primary care (given stimulus by the then emergent HIV epidemic), there was somewhat of a renaissance of interest in public health interventions, what became known as the 'New Public Health' (Berridge et al:2005). But as it turned out this was largely a false dawn. While preventative population health programmes were to be given a prominent role within the Labour Government's inequalities in health strategy (1999–2010), they were to return to the margins of state activity after 2012 in England and Wales. As Rutter et al (2017) have argued, the identification, implementation, and evaluation of effective responses to major public health challenges require a wider set of approaches than that provided through a health care system: '(A) complex systems model of public health conceptualises poor health and health inequalities as outcomes of a multitude of interdependent elements within a connected whole' (2017;2602).

Public health policy in low- and medium-income countries

Poverty and limited access to prevention programmes has chronic non-communicable disease (NCD) contributing to more than two-thirds of deaths worldwide, with 80% of these deaths occurring in low- and middle-income countries. This disproportionate share of premature death and disability only serves to exacerbate pre-existing global health inequities. It is was on this basis that the WHO Sustainable Development Goals (SDG) strategy (WHO:2015) was first developed and which has subsequently become an important stimulus for the integration of public health programmes within overall health care provision across health systems. Widening population access to prevention and treatment programmes control the population incidence of NCDs has become an essential requirement in the goal of achieving the implementation of the WHO SDGs (Niessen et al:2018;2038). The WHO has also placed a particular emphasis on cross-cutting action to end poverty and social inequality, linked to public health programmes that promote healthy lives and well-being for all at all ages. Yet it frequently remains the case that public health services and prevention programmes in many low- and medium-income countries are underfunded and not given the priority their contribution to achieving SDGs justifies. It also largely remains the case that it is the international charitable donor organisations that take the lead in determining the focus of public health programmes for child health and infectious diseases.[11] Yet by definition, these organisations operate autonomously, outside the governance mechanisms of national health healths, so their accountability to local communities will always be limited, whatever their good intentions.

An even greater challenge for public health programmes is to address the upstream causes of the double burden of disease that is typically found in low-income developing countries (LIDCs). This means investing resources to ensure the provision of clean water and the construction of modern sewage systems, sustainable employment policies, providing equitable education to 18 for all, affordable public transport systems, and access to affordable high-quality foods. It is ultimately only through these integrated social, economic, and health policies that social inequalities in health outcome can be firmly addressed.

Public health policy challenge 1: mental health in the UK

The rising numbers of people reporting mental health problems[12] in the UK is an emerging public health concern given its link with social, economic, as well as individual vulnerability factors. Yet given the psychiatric uncertainties surrounding causation, diagnosis, and prognosis, poor mental health has often been presented as an intractable problem. All too frequently, support interventions do not materialise until an individual's mental health has deteriorated to the point at which serious concerns have arisen about their personal well-being and the safety of others. It is often only then that the formal mental health care services become involved, psychiatric drug treatment and admission to a mental health facility as an inpatient may then follow. Some 8% of the total NHS budget was spent on the mental health care services in 2022–23, but this spending has risen at a slower rate than the overall rise in the NHS England budget over the past decade. It is on this basis that many have argued that mental health service funding has to increase considerably to meet rising demand, with more beds and qualified staff required (BMA:2024).

According to research produced by the Centre for Mental Health, a private research organisation commissioned by the NHS Confederation,[13] the total cost to the economy, health and care services, as well as the reduced quality of life experienced by individual's resulting from mental health issues was said to total at least £300bn in 2022.

This sum is equivalent to nearly double the current total spending budget for the NHS. The figure is broken down as follows: (a) £130bn in human costs – defined as the 'monetary value of reduced quality of life' assessed in terms of reductions in QALY scores; (b) £110bn in economic costs – these relate to the loss of tax revenues due to economic inactivity and unemployment arising from mental ill health. To this is added the costs of sickness absence, loss of productivity, and staff turnover (c) £60bn in health care costs – these relate to service provision, medication, therapy, and accommodation for people with mental health problems who are homeless (Cardoso & McHayle:2024;11).

While it is the case that not all mental health problems are preventable, especially given the uncertainties surrounding severe mental illness (SMI) characterised by psychosis and personality disorders, there is the potential to ameliorate many of the social factors that are implicated in causation through public health outreach and support programmes. The COVID-19 pandemic with its the associated lockdown and isolation is often presented as playing an important role in rising mental health disability levels. But long-standing social and economic factors such as rising material deprivation, reductions in job security, an increase in casual employment, the influence of social media impacting on personal self-esteem and identity as well as the promulgation of unrealistic expectations that predate the pandemic have also been mooted as playing an important role in the increase in reported mental health problems. Many of these factors are potentially amendable if a government has the political will to commit resources to intervening at the social and economic level.

Yet there has been only limited public health funding available via local authorities, for the development of mental health outreach programmes and facilities. What investment there has been is largely directed towards the needs of children and young people, while the provision of pubic health support services for adults of working age remains extremely limited. There have been some 'green shoots' in more recent times, one example would be local authorities (with their public health remit) working in partnership with the NHS and voluntary groups to develop what are known as 'health and well-being hubs'. The function of these neighbourhood public health hubs is to provide a single access point for support without the necessity of referral to single issue services. This service is intended for people looking for support for their mental health problems, as well as those who want to make health and lifestyle changes. Support comes through practical advice and signposting appropriate services, as well health advocacy, employment, and debt advice. There is no one 'blueprint' so a diversity of approaches adopted by different local authorities (LGA:2023). Nevertheless, given the very limited funding available for any expansion of these such initiatives remains limited.

Public health policy challenge 2: obesity in the UK

Not having a healthy weight for height has increasingly becoming the norm for adults as well as children in HIC's. Being 'overweight' is defined as having a Body Mass Index (BMI) of 30 kg/m^2 or over. Using this standardised measure, some 67% of men and 60% of women in England are deemed to be overweight or obese in total, with obesity corresponding to 26% of men and 29% of women in this group (NHS Digital:2020). This phenomenon is also apparent amongst children, with 1 in 5 children in Year 6 of Primary School (aged 10–11) being classified as obese. Perhaps surprisingly, given the historical and cultural association of obesity with wealth and over-indulgence, the gap in obesity rates between the least and most socially deprived children in Year 6 has almost doubled in a decade. Obesity is now increasingly associated with the experience of relative socio-economic inequality, with prevalence rates twice as high in the most deprived areas than the least deprived areas in England (NHS Digital:2020). Living with obesity is also associated with a lifetime higher risk of developing heart disease, stroke, diabetes, osteoarthritis, and many other associated chronic conditions. Obesity was a factor in 876,000 hospital admissions in 2019–20 (the year before the COVID-19 pandemic). This admission rate constituted an increase of 23% compared to 2017/18, and nearly 70% compared to 2015/6 (NHS Digital:2020).

The challenge of addressing these high levels of obesity is not primarily about committing more health care resources for early medical intervention. Obesity is a multifactorial condition resulting from a variety of social and economic causal pathways, and as highlighted in a research report funded by the government nearly two decades ago now, it is not amenable to a 'one-size fits all approach' (Foresight Report:2007). The social phenomenon of obesity is not an issue of volitional behaviour that can somehow be 'corrected' by individual health education in isolation from wider social interventions. Effective public health interventions require an evidence base that draws from research in the fields of the medical and life sciences as well as from policy studies and the social sciences including economics. It is this interdisciplinary understanding of the causes of obesity that has the potential to fully inform us about the range of variables in play within what has become known as the 'obesogenic environment'. The latter defined as 'the sum of influences that the surroundings, opportunities, or conditions of life have on promoting obesity in individuals or populations' (Lake & Townshend:2006).

The expression 'sum of influences' used in the quote above reflects the fact that the causal pathways that connect an individual's food consumption and their levels of physical activity are complex and not always easily delineated. However, it is possible to produce a less than exhaustive list of social, economic and cultural factors that have contributed to the emergence of the obesogenic environment in societies around the globe, these would include in no particular order the following:

- Media influences – exposure to the advertising of 'convenient' processed foods
- Affordability of processed food as opposed to healthy dietary options
- Social acceptability of 'fatness', less stigma attached to being overweight than in previous generations
- Peer Pressure – increasing prominence of an idealised body image, the unattainability of which for the majority of people is linked to the previous factor
- Loss of socio-cultural value attached to families eating, associated with a lack of parental control over children's diet
- Greater availability of 'passive home entertainment': From electronic games, social media, to good old-fashioned TV programmes
- Extension of the working day, with a lack of time for food preparation, leading to a rise in demand for convenience foods
- Rise of sedentary office (or home) working
- Reduced emphasis on physical activity in schools because of the demands of an exam-led national curriculum Linked to decline in numbers of those actively participating in sport and exercise over a lifetime

- Greater urbanisation leading to a reduction in the space available for physical activities
- Reliance on powered vehicles for even short journeys
- Walking and cycling to work and school remains challenging due to exclusive car-friendly urban planning

Interventions to promote so-called healthy lifestyles will always be constrained by the broader social structural and material realities of life in a consumer society where even routinised daily activities such as eating and exercising are shaped by the marketisation of commodities. Any public health strategy designed to reduce the levels of obesity in society has to be both systematic and integrated. Systematic, in the sense of understanding the interplay that occurs between a range of socio-cultural factors. Integrated, in the sense that focusing only at the level of health care interventions and health education initiatives would be to ignore the crucial role that social and economic policy can play in promoting affordable healthy food consumption, exercise, and physical play. There is also the potential for local authorities to involve neighbourhood communities in contributing to the redesign of their shared urban environment in order to make physical activities such as walking and cycling safe and inclusive. This can give communities a stake in their future health, rather than being the subject of imposed schemes, which often produce resentment at perceived 'nanny statism'.

Notes

1 Following the classic work of Jürgen Habermas (1962), the distinction between the public and civil spheres of society (with the private sphere constituted by family, home and individual life constituting a third sphere) is one that identifies civil society as the sphere of 'commodity exchange and social labour', and the public sphere as constituted through the activities of those institutions constitutive of the 'political realm'. Habermas himself recognised that the distinction between these 'spheres' was increasingly being blurred. Some 60 years later, this process is now fully advanced to the point that it is often difficult to find any distinction between the public, civic, and private.
2 The concept of the 'ideal-type' is discussed in Chapter 2.
3 *Absolute* measures of inequality measure the *differences* in rates of mortality, typically between the highest and lowest socio-economic groups, while *relative* measures assess the change in the distribution of the rate of mortality measured as a *ratio* between socio-economic groups in a population.
4 The 'inverse care law' was first described by Julian Tudor Hart in 1971, and states that, 'the availability of good medical care tends to vary *inversely* with the need for it in the population served'.
5 Discussed in Chapter 7.
6 This local authority public health funding does not include epidemiological population surveillance, immunisation services, disease prevention programmes, and the operation of public health laboratories (much of this work has subsequently been outsourced to the private sector), the responsibility for which remains with the Department of Health. It also excludes government funding for public health research as well as health-related public works such as sewage treatment, pollution abatement, and clean water supplies.
7 Discussed in Chapter 5 in relation to the 'efficiency' of health systems.
8 The concept of institutional path-dependency was introduced in Chapter 2.
9 The influence of the medical profession within the newly founded NHS was discussed in Chapter 3.
10 Local authorities retained some their health protection functions.

11 The issues surrounding the delivery of public health policy in both Ghana and Kenya were discussed in Chapter 6.
12 MIND, the UK mental health charity utilise the expression, 'mental health problems' and this is the phrase that will be adopted here. MIND state on their webpage: 'that many people have told us this phrase feels helpful for them. But you might be familiar with terms such as "poor emotional health", "overload", "burnt out" or "overwhelmed". Or you may feel that terms such as "mental illness" or "mental health issues" describe your experiences better' (MIND:2024).
13 The NHS Confederation is representative body or membership association for NHS institutions, specifically senior management in those institutions. It is not part of the structure of the NHS itself.

References

Acheson, D (1998) *Independent Inquiry into Inequalities in Health*. London. The Stationery Office.
Berridge, V and Loughlin, K (2005) Smoking and the new health education in Britain 1950s–1970s, *American Journal of Public Health*, vol. 95, no. 6, 956–964.
BMA – British Medical Association (2024) *Mental Health Pressures in England*. www.bma.org.uk (accessed 04/2024).
Cardoso, F and McHayle, Z (2024) *The Economic and Social Costs of Mental Ill Health*. London. Centre for Mental Health.
Department of Health (1999) *Saving Lives: Our Healthier Nation*. Cm 4386. London. HMSO.
Department of Health (2003) *Tackling Health Inequalities: A Programme for Action*. London. DH.
Department of Health (2009) *Tackling Health Inequalities: 10 Years On. A Review of Developments in Tackling Health Inequalities in England Over the Last 10 Years*. London. DH.
Department of Health and Social Security (1979) *Inequalities in Health: Report of a Research Working Group*. London. DHSS.
Foresight Report (2007) *Tackling obesities – Future choices project*. London. Department of Innovation, Universities and Skills, The Stationary Office.
FPH – Faculty of Public Health (2020) *Functions and Standards of a Public Health System*. https://www.fph.org.uk/ (accessed 09/2022).
Habermas, J (1962 trans 1989) *The Structural Transformation of the Public Sphere and Deliberative Politics*. Cambridge. Polity.
Health and Social Care Act (2012) https://legislation.gov.uk/ (accessed 01/2023).
Health Foundation (2024) *Investing in the Public Health Grant*. www.health.org.uk (accessed 04/2024).
Lake, A and Townshend, T (2006) Obesogenic environments: exploring the built and food environments, *Journal of the Royal Society for the Promotion of Health*, vol. 126, no. 6, 262–267.
LGA – Local Government Association (2023) *Health and Wellbeing Hubs: Delivering local services under one roof*. www.local.gov.uk (accessed 02/2024).
Martin, S, Lomas, J and Claxton, K (2020) Is an ounce of prevention worth a pound of cure? A cross-sectional study of the impact of English public health grant on mortality and morbidity, *BMJ Open*, vol. 10, e036411.
MIND (2024) *Different perspectives on mental health and mental illness*. https://mind.org.uk (accessed 04/2024).
NHS Digital (2020) *Statistics on obesity, physical activity and diet: England 2020*. https://digital.nhs.uk/data-and-information/publications (accessed 03/2021).
Niessen, L, Mohan, D, Akuoku, J, Mirelman, A, Ahmed, S, Koehlmoos, T, Trujillo, A, Khan, J and Peters, D (2018) Tackling socioeconomic inequalities and non-communicable diseases in low-income and middle-income countries under the sustainable development agenda, *The Lancet*, vol. 391, no. 10134, 2036–2046.
Office of National Statistics (2023) *Local authority revenue expenditure and financing: 2023–24 budget, England*. www.gov.uk (accessed 03/2024).

Parkhurst, J and Abeysinghe, S (2016) What constitutes "good" evidence for public health and social policy-making? From hierarchies to appropriateness, *Social Epistemology*, vol. 30: 665–679.

Rutter, H et al (2017) The need for a complex systems model of evidence for public health, *The Lancet*, vol. 390, 2602–2604.

World Health Organisation (2015) *Sustainable Development Goals.* www.who.int (accessed 10/2022).

World Health Organisation (2022) *Essential Public Health Functions: A Sustainable approach to ensure multi-sectoral actions for population health.* www.who.int (accessed 02/24).

CHAPTER 10

The challenge of constructing a pharmaceutical policy

The 'post-genomic revolution'

The decade-long Human Genome Project (HGP), an international research collaboration to sequence the whole human genome, was finally completed in 2003. When the original funding for the HGP was announced back in 1990, it was claimed that sequencing the human genome would provide the information that would enable clinical practice to move from an era of 'mass health' to the individual 'customisation' of medicine (Dumit:2012;8). This 'post-genomic revolution' as it was subsequently termed, had been expected to open the possibilities for linking the associations found to exist between genetic variants and disease risk in order to construct individualised 'genome profiles'. However, when the HGP was completed it produced the finding that there were only approximately 20,000 human genes, about the same number as in a starfish, rather than the anticipated finding of a 'gene-for' every human outcome, understanding the relationship between genetics and disease had just became even more complex.

As it began to be recognised that significant genotype variation occurred across populations, so it was realised that it would be necessary to establish SNP[1] databases in order to gain a purchase on individual variability and predisposition to disease. Once the databases began to be built they opened up the possibilities for genome-wide association studies (GWAS). GWAS are in principle hypothesis-free methods that seek to examine SNPs across the genome in the study of common but complex diseases, where many genetic variations can contribute to an individual's risk of that disease. GWAS constitute the potential database for genomic profiling, able to link microbiological information (genotype) with the social and medical history (identifiable 'risk' factors) of an individual. Over the following decade, billions of research dollars were spent on GWAS, but this research has identified a disappointingly low number of gene variants of genuine significance for human health given the initially high level of expectation (Tutton:2016;1). Even by 2010, it was clear that in order to achieve the translational goals of utilising genomic information for future clinical diagnostic and therapeutic interventions it would be necessary to scale up research programmes to sequence the genomic make-up of hundreds of thousands of individuals. Subsequently, mass sequencing programmes were set up in a number of national settings, some of these have focused on single diseases, while others have been more broad-based.

Genomics England was established by the Department of Health in 2013 with a budget of £300 million and tasked with the goal of sequencing 100,000 genomes from National Health Service (NHS) patients and their families, who were living with a

DOI: 10.4324/9781003564249-14

rare disease, as well as patients with common cancers. One of the explicit targets of this data collection programme was to kick start the development of a UK genomics industry. NHS England established 13 genomics medical centres specifically to identify, enrol, and gain consent from participants in the project. The genomic data that was subsequently collected and analysed was linked to the patient's health records in partnership with NHS Digital, the health information arm of the NHS, and made available to researchers and the genomic pharmaceutical industries via the UK Biobank.[2] The latter had been established in 2006 as an initiative jointly funded by the Department of Health and the Medical Research Council (part of the UK government funded Research and Innovation agency – UKRI), together with the medical research charity, the Welcome Trust. Similar initiatives were also established in the three other devolved countries of the UK. The target of sequencing 100,000 genomes was successfully achieved in December 2018.

The USA was slightly behind the curve in establishing a similar research programme to the UK. It was not until 2015 that President Barack Obama made the announcement that the USA would embark on a government-funded initiative under the auspices of the federal health care research agency, the National Institutes of Health (NIH), entitled the *All of Us Program*. The objective was to enrol over one million participants who would be expected to share their genomic and health behavioural data generated or captured over a period of ten years or more. This data would be sourced from sequencing programmes, electronic medical records, personally reported information, and digital health technologies. The anticipated outcome of this programme was not only to drive the understanding of disease biology and pathogenesis, but to constitute the informational basis for developing 'precision-driven' health care for individuals and populations (Ginsburg & Philips:2018;694). The programme finally opened for enrolment in May 2018, and as of February 2024, more than 750,000 participants had enrolled and contributed their 'biospecimens' (NIH:2024).

Back in the UK, following the successful meeting of the 100,000 sequencing target in 2018, the government announced plans to expand the programme to sequence 500,000 whole genomes within five years. In order to achieve this ambitious new target, a public-private consortium was established to partner with the UK Biobank. This consortium involved commercial biotech companies as well as four large pharmaceutical companies, Amgen, AstraZeneca, GlaxoSmithKline, and Johnson & Johnson. This consortium together contributed £230 million of funding over the five years of the project (UK Biobank:2024). The half a million genome sequencing programme was completed in 2023 and it clearly demonstrated the commitment of the UK government to invest in the future of genomic research.

Yet the question arises as to what were the key drivers of this significant public-private collaborative undertaking? Was the primary concern solely to establish a national genomic database to facilitate the translation of genomic research into viable clinical interventions through a process of patient risk assessment, diagnosis, and treatment that would then be freely available in the NHS? Or did the strategy have the equally compelling objective of developing the UK Biobank as an infrastructural resource for the construction of a life sciences-orientated industrial strategy? The latter was after all the model that had been followed in the USA for decades. The US government-funded NIH has channelled tens of billions of dollars of public money into early stage translational medical research and development, this including the funding of the HGP to the tune of $3 billion. Without this state involvement it is unlikely that the pharmaceutical and medical technology market on its own would not have generated the necessary investment given the uncertainties associated with the outcomes of medical research. For example, one study has found that of the 200 medicines approved in the USA between 2010 and 2016, NIH-funded research had played a role in the development of every one of them (Cleary et al:2018, cited in Dearden:2023;91).

Promissory visions: pharmacogenomics and clinical medicine

As Richard Tutton noted over a decade ago, 'personalised' or 'precision'[3] medicine is a particularly pertinent example of the high expectations engendered by the much hyped 'genomic revolution' described above: '(I)t encapsulates both the excesses of promissory science and the inevitable disappointments and disputes that follow. Those who were once hopeful or excited in the 1990s by the prospects of what would be achieved by genomics are now less certain .... (P)ersonalised medicine is therefore an appealing yet ambiguous and contested term and is as such an ideal one for engaging with the claims and counterclaims about the value of genomics to biomedicine' (Tutton:2014;3). When sociologists such as Tutton use the term 'promissory science', they are pointedly referring to the situation that arises when, 'novel technologies and fundamental changes in scientific principle do not substantively pre-exist themselves, except and only in terms of the imaginings, expectations and visions that have shaped their potential' (Borup et al:2006;285). Generating positive expectations about the predicted benefits of scientific research, in this case in the field of genomic medicine, are seen to be an absolute requirement in securing the support of government and major commercial funders necessary to translate and implement the research into everyday clinical practice.

In the post-HGP period, despite or maybe because of its promissory elements, significant progress has been made in the field of pharmacogenomics (PGx) concerned with the understanding of the role of the individual human genome in drug response. Advances in PGx have enhanced the ability to identify DNA variants that have the potential to alter the absorption, distribution, metabolism, and excretion of a prescribed drug (known as *pharmacokinetics*) in an individual, as well as influencing the effect of that drug (known as *pharmacodynamics*), either directly on a targeted organ or indirectly on other tissues or on the immune mechanisms of that individual (Swift:2022;175). The promissory claim for scaled-up routine pre-emptive clinical PGx testing is that it will be able to identify DNA variations in a particular patient's genetic background that would indicate the possibility of potential adverse drug reactions (ADRs). ADRs were the primary cause of 6% of all patient admissions within the NHS in 2014, and equated to 4% of hospital bed capacity at that time (RPS:2014). In 2018, one report estimated that avoidable ADRs consumed 181,626 bed-days in the NHS, a direct cause in 712 deaths, and contributing to a further 1,708 deaths (Elliott et al:2018). On the basis of a patient's PGx information, a clinician will in principle be able to prescribe the most effective and safest drug for that individual.

These promissory claims for the clinical benefits of integrating a PGx-informed patient management system within a health care service have been enhanced by the further claim (from leading biotech and pharmaceutical companies as well as many academic researchers) that a PGx testing and prescribing system will bring with it significant reductions in health care expenditure through early prevention. For example, cancer surveillance has traditionally been predicated on tumour anatomic location and histology reports, but with the application of molecular markers such as gene expression profiles, the promise is that heterogeneous population subgroups associated with different risk factors and treatment responses can be identified (Khoury et al 2022;1634). In private insurance-based health care systems such as that of the USA, the ability to effectively reduce ADRs has the potential to reduce an individual's health insurance premiums. Less positively, it could also mean that the identification of individual members of sub-groups at greatest health risk could be the basis for denying insurance cover.

Integrating genomic medicine within health care systems

Despite the promissory claims for a PGx-based clinical practice discussed above, there remain significant challenges to be overcome if genomic medicine is to become a viable mainstream proposition for health care provision in the future. The barriers to widespread adoption, 'span diverse domains, including data integration and interpretation, workforce capacity and capability, public acceptability and government engagement, paucity of evidence for clinical utility and cost-effectiveness, and ethical and legislative issues' (Stark et al:2019;13).

One of the key challenges for individual drug prescribing that requires prior diagnostic genomic testing (known as 'combined treatment') rather than the standardised 'one size fits all' approach that is the norm within health care systems, is the much higher costs associated with this pre-emptive method. If combined treatment was to be routinely offered in primary care settings, then it has been estimated that around four million people would have to be subject to annual genomic testing in the UK (Youssef et al:2021). On this basis, some have argued that universal pre-emptive testing is not a practical proposition for the NHS and that some form of eligibility criteria should be introduced: '(T)his may involve prioritizing patients based on other risk factors. Limiting testing to situations where high doses are indicated, or to medicines associated with the most severe or common adverse drug reactions' (Magavern et al:2021;4550). In practice, the primary target for PGx combined therapies are those groups of high-risk patients living with a known genetic disorder; this is a relatively small number in terms of the total number of people receiving treatment in the NHS. Combination pharmaceutical therapies would never constitute a mass market equivalent to the 'one size fits all' blockbuster drugs that constitute the primary source of revenue and profit for the large pharmaceutical corporations. This in turn raises the issue of the commitment of these companies to develop and deliver these PGx therapeutics at an affordable cost for an NHS (Crinson:2021;89).

The second key challenge is to determine the most effective strategy for integrating the benefits of genomic-based medicine into the NHS without undermining its key principles of universalism and equity. Integration would require an expansion of existing health information systems, and specifically '(T)he curation of the pharmacogenomic evidence, expert design of the pharmacogenomic test, curation of predicted consequences of the genetic variants, clinical expertise regarding drug prescribing and alternatives, and technical expertise to support laboratory testing, reporting, and decision support' (Roden et al:2019;528). This investment would come at considerable cost and at a time when the NHS is already struggling to meet the rising demand for health care.

Some form of consequentialist priority-setting strategy[4] for access to combined therapies might well be inevitable. In private insurance-based health systems such as the USA, the issue of equity of provision is even starker. As a recent US review noted: '(I)f genomics and precision medicine are to improve health for all, generational inequities embedded in society at large and the US health system have to be acknowledged and addressed. Any success resulting from a siloed equity approach to genomics could be overshadowed by other poor health outcomes unless the underlying determinants of health inequities, such as the lack of access to health care, healthy food, air, and water; inadequate housing; chronic stress; and exposures to environmental toxins are addressed. Together with core drivers such as structural racism' (Khoury et al:2022;1633).

A third challenge is how to overcome the current limited level of clinician knowledge around genomics and the efficacy of PGx therapies in order to facilitate their application in everyday General Practice. The majority of practising doctors in the UK have received little to no teaching of the principles of genomic medicine while at medical school. Medical expertise in clinical pharmacogenomics remains the exception in both primary and secondary care settings and mostly confined to relatively few academic-led health care institutions (Magavern:2021;4550). An allied consideration is the on-going development of new genomic medical technologies and treatments that make it a challenge for many doctors to stay update: 'Although the scientific evidence and clinical benefit of PGx is strong, it can all remain unclear due to poor literacy in genomics, which lowers the overall acceptance' (Krebs & Milani:2019;6). While some may point to an inherent culture of professional resistance when it comes to embracing new forms of clinical practice, this would be an unfair comment. Many doctors, particularly in primary care, continue to have serious concerns about the lack of clear evidence for the efficaciousness of PGx sequencing and testing for individual patients as part of everyday clinical prescribing (Rafi et al:2020).

Furthermore, there are also widespread concerns, not limited to members of the medical profession, about the practicality of imposing a radical change in patient management within the current health system. This is the view that without a commensurate increase in public investment in health care staffing, professional training, and the introduction of the a more expansive and accessible national health information infrastructure, the 'genomic revolution' as applied to health care could falter. In 2022, a joint working party that included the Royal College of Physicians and the British Pharmacological Society examined the implications of PGx for clinical prescribing in the future and identified a range of factors that constituted an 'unmet need for planned, systematic implementation and training' (Swift:2022;174). The final report recommended the adoption of 'an iterative developmental strategy'. This strategy would include a thorough-going identification of planning priorities, a review of the most optimal form of genetic testing for patients, and an integrated approach to patient genomic data reporting via electronic patient records consistent across primary and secondary care. Most significantly of all, the joint report recommended, 'a UK NHS-wide centrally-funded, equitable service, enabling long-term patient follow-up, targeting the most clinically cost-effective gene-drug pairs, monitoring delivery standards and thereby delivering maximum long-term efficiency' (Swift:2022;176). As of 2024, the NHS in England has made no significant progress on developing a strategy that addresses these essential requirements.

Unsurprisingly, given the limited availability of resources, the integration of GPx medical interventions within low- and medium-income developing countries is even less advanced than in health systems in HICs. A degree of scepticism can also be detected in terms of the perceived value-for-money benefits of a wholesale application of PGx approaches within these under-resourced health systems. This view is evident in the following account set out in a recent systematic review of the cost-effectiveness of PGx in developing counties: 'The adoption of pharmacogenomics in the healthcare system has economic consequences to patients, payers, and the pharmaceutical industry due to the cost pharmacogenomics testing, cost of drugs, and additional costs to conduct clinical trials to validate the biomarkers. Therefore the economic impact of pharmacogenomics testing should be critically evaluated before the practice can be implemented' (Sukri et al:2022;148). The conclusion of this systematic review regarding the cost-effectiveness of PGx was mixed. There was some evidence in support of its application as an effective treatment for certain selected diseases such as certain cancers and cardiovascular issues, but not in relation to ADRs and epilepsy. The conclusion of the review was that given the relative paucity of GWAS conducted amongst populations in the developing regions of the globe, there was just too little evidence available to systematically evaluate the cost-effectiveness of PGx applications for patient care (Sukri:2022;157). It should be added that this was a designed as a clinical review and as such did not take into account the wider health policy concerns of the costs and funding required to integrate PGx into routine practice within these developing health systems.

'Big Pharma' and its role in the development of genomic-based medicine

It might be supposed that the large multinational pharmaceutical corporations ('Big Pharma') would have played an active role in the development of PGx clinical applications and in promoting their uptake across health care systems, but this has not been the case. As of early 2024, the American Federal Drug Administration (FDA) had published PGx biomarker labelling information for some 500 previously approved pharmaceutical drugs (FDA:2024). The objective in updating product labels with DNA variant information on already marketed drugs (in some instances decades after first approval) is to make the prescribing of these drugs safer and more effective for patients based on the ability to pre-emptively test them for DNA variants. Yet relatively few next-generation combination PGx therapies have been developed by pharmaceutical companies in recent years and subsequently been approved by the FDA. This poses legitimate questions about the economic business model adopted by pharmaceutical companies that places profitability before health need in their drug research development and commercial investment decisions. What are the factors that have led to the situation where pharmaceutical companies are not investing at the level one might expect given the apparent opportunities of this new science for developing new products?

Here the impact of the process known as 'financialisation' on corporate strategic investment decision-making is key. Financialisation[5] has previously been discussed in the context of the changing relationship between national states and global financial markets from the late 1980s onwards and which ultimately was seen as having a devastating impact on national fiscal policy following the banking and financial crash of 2008. The process of financialisation has also played an important role in re-shaping the business strategies of the non-banking sectors of the economy, in particular Big Pharma, a development that was assisted in no small part by the limited regulatory role played by national governments in the globalised financial marketplace. As Nick Dearden explains, in his polemical account entitled *Pharmanomics*: '(W)hereas in the past a drug company was primarily competing against other drug companies to make profitable medicines, in the modern economy drug companies are competing against all profit-making enterprises – whether they make cars, biscuits or financial services ... they are not judged by the standard of the product they make, but by the short-term returns their operations can generate for their investors. If higher profits come from trading derivatives, or buying up and asset-stripping other companies, or trading your own shares to keep your stock high, so be it' (2023;44). In recent years, the financial returns to pharmaceutical company shareholders have actually exceeded the profits made by these companies. One study of two UK-based Big Pharma companies listed on the stock market, GlaxoSmithKline (GSK) and AstraZeneca, found that they returned over 100% of their net income to shareholders in 2020 (Haslem et al:2021 – cited in Dearden:2023;47). While in the USA, between 2016 and 2020, 14 of the top Big Pharma companies spent $577 billion on stock buybacks and shareholder dividends, this equated to $56 billion more than they collectively spent of research and development (Moore:2021 – cited in Dearden:2023;57).

One particular outcome of the logic of financialisation was a series of mergers and acquisitions that reduced the overall number of pharmaceutical companies worldwide, but increased in the size of those that remained. By the second decade of this century, just 10 Big Pharma companies constituted around 90% of the total global turnover of the industry. While the 27 largest pharmaceutical companies (assessed in terms of market capitalisation) together held financial reserves of $237 billion, the top ten held more than 60% of this total. It was primarily the cash flows acquired through the process of financialisation, rather than profits derived from their core pharmaceutical production business, that were used to amass these significant financial reserves, but these reserves have not invested in productive capacity. Accompanying this accumulation of financial reserves was a seemingly counter-intuitive concomitant increase in debt, with the top ten Big Pharma companies seeing their collective debt rising from $50 billion to $310 billion in the period 2000–18 (Fernandez & Klinge:2020;19–21). This acquisition of debt by Big Pharma was a direct outcome of the cheap credit that was obtainable from banks and other financial institutions from the late 1990s onwards. It was used to bankroll the process of financialisation, subsidising the difference between the profits of a company and the need to increase shareholder dividends. High levels of easily obtainable credit were also used to gain leverage in order to buy out and acquire smaller competitor companies. All this borrowing enabled the Big Pharma companies to be become even bigger, enriching existing shareholders and attracting further investors. But funding investment through debt is not sustainable over the long term. For many of these corporations the strategy of financialisation continues in lieu of greater productivity in their core business: 'Big Pharma spends more and more of its resources trying to bolster the value of its intangible assets, rather than engaging in productive activity ... turning (them) into hedge funds with pharmaceutical companies attached' (Dearden:2023;53).

As Dearden goes on to explain, 'that so much money is chasing proportionally less research and fewer drugs explains why the price of medicine has increased so much. It is not to do with the cost of making the drugs – in fact, medicine prices are entirely unrelated to research costs; rather it is hard-wired into the financialisation of the industry' (2023;49). The recent history of Big Pharma R&D expenditure is characterised not so much by bringing on-stream innovative new medicines to address on-going and emergent disease across the globe, but more about making only marginal changes to existing medicines in order to extend their patents. This R&D strategy brings substantial profits to companies with little financial risk. Big Pharma also often buy-up the right to produce medicines that smaller companies have developed through investment in research. As a direct consequence, since 1999, the average profit margin of Big Pharma companies has increased exponentially, some three times the average profit margin of corporations found in other industries (Hawksbee et al:2022 – cited in Dearden:2023;64).

This shift in the core business strategy of Big Pharma is particularly well illustrated by the low priority that has been attached to developing new vaccines to meet the rising demand for infectious disease management. The production of vaccines was once a key staple for pharmaceutical companies, but they have always been a risky investment because of the high R&D costs involved and the low profit margins. Usually, only a single dose of a vaccine is required (with the occasional booster) to immunise an individual, in contrast to the long-term consumption of block buster medicines developed for chronic conditions. In 2018, only 1% of global Big Pharma R&D spending was invested in emerging infectious diseases (Dearden:2023;89). The lack of vaccine-preparedness for a pandemic such as COVID-19 clearly demonstrated where the interests of Big Pharma lie. In the spring of 2020 as the extent of the spread of COVID-19 became rapidly apparent, the US government was required to invest £18 billion of public money in order to incentivise Big Pharma to start researching, trialling, and producing vaccines. This was combined with its commitment to buy all the effective vaccine that could be produced, in what was entitled 'Operation Warp Speed'.

Yet the breakthrough in developing the first effective vaccines came not from within the Big Pharma corporations, but from a biotech company called Moderna. This company had no products on the market prior to the pandemic, and like most biotech companies operated on the basis of selling its translational R&D to Big Pharma for up-scaled production and marketisation. Yet in the case of COVID-19, the company was able to draw on its genomic research know-how to develop a molecular-based approach to vaccine development. This research utilised the known attributes of a messenger RNA (mRNA) corresponding to a viral protein in order to trigger a normal immune response, rather than relying on the traditional method of developing vaccines using part of an actual bacteria or virus. This biotechnology required no large factories to grow virus cultures, mRNA vaccines could be produced cheaply and quickly in laboratory conditions. The mRNA technology was also adaptable, enabling vaccines to be modified to take account of the inevitable mutation of the virus. Moderna's vaccine reportedly took a weekend to design (Dearden:2023;95).

Astra Zeneca, an Anglo-Swiss corporation, was the other main industry contributor to developing a COVID-19 vaccine, and like Moderna, was also untypical of many of its Big Pharma competitors. In the decade preceding the pandemic, Astra Zeneca had begun to shift its growth strategy away from the path of financialisation. This change in its investment policy was not necessarily driven by a return to core business principles, but rather had been forced on the company as a result of a number of expensive legal rulings. As its blockbuster drugs neared the end of their patent monopolies, Astra Zeneca had attempted to misuse its dominant position to force producers of generic copies of its products out of the market. It was subsequently found guilty of abusing its market position by the European Court of Justice in 2012. Two years earlier in the USA, it had been found guilty of illegally marketing an antipsychotic drug for uses that were not approved by the FDA as being safe and effective. On the basis of these charges, the company agreed to a $520 million settlement paid to the US government. In the same year the company was also forced to agree to pay a £505 million settlement to the UK Inland Revenue after being found to have committed a 15-year series of tax-dodges. Following these rulings, the company began to move to end their stock pay-back programmes and began to invest in R&D for new medicines (Dearden:2023;132). Significantly, Astra Zeneca's investment in the development of an effective COVID-19 vaccine was only achieved following its partnering with the Jenner Institute at the University of Oxford. The Jenner Institute's ground-breaking R&D work having been publically funded by the British Government to the tune of £67 million, with additional charitable funding.

The long-term impact of adopting the financialisation model was further evident in the conduct of Big Pharma during the height of the COVID-19 pandemic. At this time, pressure was being placed on governments to temporarily suspend Big Pharma's intellectual property (IP) rights over their COVID-19 vaccines, in order to allow national pharmaceutical producers in medium- and low-income countries to manufacture their own vaccines at cost. Health systems in these countries desperately needed to make up the shortfall in vaccines supplied by Big Pharma who were accused of stockpiling in order to keep prices high. The response of these international corporations was to spend millions of dollars lobbying both the US government and the European Commission to resist any waver of their existing patents, spending at the very minimum some €36 million to influence the European Commission decision, overriding the EU lobby transparency rules in doing so (Corporate Europe Observatory:2021).

In summary, the long-term outcome of Big Pharma's adoption of a business model shaped by the imperatives of financialisation is their questionable commitment to the development of new PGx combined therapeutics, as well as vaccines, for routine application within clinical medical practice. Without the corporate investment necessary to scale up personalised genomic-based drug applications, the promise of this evolving field to bring about more effective clinical management of patients will be stymied. It remains the case that for the majority of Big Pharma companies ensuring high yield returns to their shareholders is their number one priority, while meeting the requirements of national health care systems for more cost-effective treatment therapies often comes in a poor second.

'The Elephant in the Room': the governance of UK pharmaceutical policy

The role of the state in balancing the infrastructural and profitability requirements of the pharmaceutical industry while ensuring that it meets the requirements of the NHS for new safe and cost-effective medicines is a crucial one. The successful achievement of these two objectives is in essence what constitutes a 'pharmaceutical policy'.

The UK government's pharmaceutical policy reflects the core objectives of its industrial and economic strategy, that is, to improve the infrastructure, the research knowledge base for innovation, and the technical skills that are 'crucial for economic growth, boosting productivity and competitiveness' (HM Treasury:2021). Over the past decade, and specifically in relation to the pharmaceutical industry, the government's strategy has been focused on ensuring that: '(T)he UK is a favourite location for businesses to research, develop and market new products. The ultimate aim is to encourage investment in the UK life sciences sector to grow the economy' (Naci & Forrest:2023;11). But in return, a pharmaceutical policy must also guarantee that in return for the public investment in essential infrastructure, financial incentives, and the training of the next generation of bioscientists, the pharmaceutical industry meets the requirements of the NHS for cost-effective and efficacious therapeutic products.

What is termed the 'core biopharmaceutical sector'[6] has in recent years been one of the strongest-performing industrial sectors in the UK, and the support provided by the government has been a key contributory factor in its productivity and growth. It is widely acknowledged that public funding of early stage R&D, including clinical trials and national programmes such as the UK Biobank 100,000 genome sequencing research (described above), 'has a disproportionately large effect on the development of drugs that offer meaningful therapeutic benefits' (Naci & Forrest:2023;20). In 2021/22, the core biopharmaceutical sector generated £46 billion in turnover and employing 70,000 people. This accounted for 43% of the total turnover of the life sciences sector of the economy. 2021/22 was also the sixth consecutive year of growth in turnover and a rise in employment within this sector of industry (ONS:2024c).

Nevertheless, for Big Pharma, the UK remains a relatively small market constituting just 3% of global sales in 2021. In the same year, Europe as a whole (including the UK) contributed 23% of the market value of global sales, while the North American market accounted for a 49% share (EFPIA:2022). It is the market incentives offered by the US health system that is key for Big Pharma profitability. The US health system, characterised 'by a fragmented payer landscape that allows companies to charge higher prices, that drives global R&D for Big Pharma ... (T)his results in health systems in other parts of the world, including the UK, approving and paying for products that were primarily designed for the US market' (Naci & Forrest:2023;11). This overriding focus on the US health market is one of the major reasons why the incentives offered by the UK government have only a limited impact on the product development investment decisions of Big Pharma. Furthermore, UK government pharmaceutical policy can be seen as characterised by the conflicting priorities of multiple government departments. These include not only the Department of Health and Social Care (DHSC), but also the Department for Business, Energy and Industrial Strategy (BEIS). The 'Office for Life Sciences (OLS), sits between the DHSC and BEIS and also plays a pivotal role in shaping the UK pharmaceutical policy landscape in recent years (Naci & Forrest:2023;13).

Governance[7] is the umbrella term that covers all those organisational process that are concerned to ensure the transparency and public accountability of decision-making and resource allocation within a health care system. This includes the establishment of regulatory mechanisms and guidelines to moderate and control the effective and efficient performance of that system. In relation to medicines, regulatory mechanisms exist to ensure that prescribed medicines are safe and efficient. All prescribed therapeutic drugs in the UK were until 2020, subject to approval via the European Medicines Agency (EMA). This body coordinates the regulatory assessment of all new medicines conducted by national agencies across the EU, and until January 2020 when the UK formally left the EU included the UK Medicines and HealthCare Products Regulatory Agency (MHRA). After the UK left the EU, the MHRA became the standalone medicines approving agency. The assessment process itself involves evaluating the safety and efficacy data derived from clinical trials and provides the risk-benefit information necessary for clinical use.

The UK also has an additional level of regulatory control for the approval of new medicines, this is concerned with assessing their cost-effectiveness for use in the NHS. This role is performed by an arms-length body that was first established in 1999, the National Institute of Clinical Excellence (NICE).[8] NICE is responsible for coordinating what is termed Health Technology Assessments (HTAs) that determine the relative cost-effectiveness of all MHRA approved (for safety and efficacy only) medicines utilising the QALY cost-utility formula. NICE therefore plays an important role in regulating the clinical demand for pharmaceuticals. It has the authority to exclude drugs that fall below the threshold of cost-effectiveness from the approved NHS prescribing list, this list is incorporated within the clinical practice guidelines that doctors in the NHS are required to follow in their patient management decision-making. The NHS medicines governance system also incentives to 'reward' the cost-effective prescribing practice of General Practitioners in primary care settings; this system of incentives is managed through the Quality Outcomes framework (QOF).[9]

But NHS governance mechanisms aside, there are clear limits to the ability of the UK government to control pharmaceutical product pricing or to incentivise Big Pharma investment in the R&D of those therapeutic products that will meet the requirements of the NHS. Big Pharma are autonomous organisations that determine the direction of their own R&D investment, production, supply, and the ultimately the cost of their products. Attempts to impose restraints that may serve to limit profit maximisation are frequently successfully countered by Big Pharma through its lobbying power and ability to influence government pharmaceutical policy at the highest levels. Big Pharma operates a legal system of payments to health care organisations and to doctors (although limited by the NHS regulations on cost-effective prescribing), they also often provide financial support to patient advocacy groups (PAGs). Pharmaceutical companies have a clear interest in persuading these PAGs that their products are efficacious, however high their cost. Although PAGs have a marginal position within the formal regulatory processes undertaken by NICE, their views frequently command a legitimacy within the court of wider public and political opinion. Getting these PAGs onside is also important for the companies as they themselves are prevented from legally advertising their prescription drugs directly to the consumer market.

The activities undertaken by Big Pharma companies to protect their market position and promote their products typically operate, following Steven Lukes' model of power (1974/2004),[10] at the third latent 'dimension' where power is manifest as 'the corruption of communication'. As summarised by the ethicist Andrew Edgar: '(B)ig Pharma has every right to pursue legitimate sales and profits. In order to protect patients and the general public, this pursuit is already highly regulated. No organisation or institution holds absolute power. However, it has been argued that this overt regulation, at the first or second dimension of power, in creating the peculiar environment of the pharmaceutical market, has led to third dimensional power responses by the industry. Power is expressed in the shaping of certain conceptions of the patient-consumer, in disease-mongering and in distorting public debate over resource prioriti-sation' (Edgar:2013;303).

Over the last two decades, and despite the existence of cost-effectiveness regula-tory process, the annual cost to the NHS in England of prescribing in hospitals and the community has increased at a faster rate than the growth in the annual budget of NHS England. In 2004–05, the cost of list price medicines was £10.3 billion (NHS Digital:2005) while public expenditure on the NHS in England that year was £75 billion (HM Treasury:2005), equating to approximately 13.7% of total NHS spend-ing. Fifteen years later in 2019–20 (the year prior to the COVID-19 pandemic), the cost of list price medicines was now £21 billion (NHS Digital:2020), while expendi-ture for the NHS in England was £122 billion (NHS England:2020), equating to approximately 17.2% of total NHS spending. In 2021, the NHS introduced a new accounting methodology that used the actual costs paid by hospitals for pharmaceu-ticals, including any negotiated discounts, rather than the industry's own list price cost of medicines, which had been the case in the published data up until then. The apparent reduction in NHS prescribing costs since this date is attributable to these changes in accounting. In 2022–23, the cost of medicines paid by NHS in England was £18.5 billion (NHSBSA:2023).

The UK spends less on prescribed medicines both in real terms (per capita) and in relative terms (both as a percentage of Total Health Spending and as a percentage of GDP) than the average for OECD member countries. But an exponential rise in the cost in pharmaceuticals over the past decade is evident. In part this reflects the increasing prevalence of chronic conditions linked to an ageing population, combined with social and environmental factors that have contributed to this burden of disease. Yet despite this expansion in demand for their products, the model of financialisation adopted by Big Pharma will always seek to maximise profit over the affordability of medicines in all health care systems (Dearden:2023;56).

Notes

1 Single nucleotide polymorphisms (SNP) are the most common type of genetic variation and occur normally throughout a person's DNA. These variations may be unique or occur in many individuals, and it is on that understanding that more than 100 million SNPs have been found in populations around the world.
2 There are many types of biobanks (with the UK Biobank being just one example), but they can be broadly defined as any collection or 'biorepository' of human biological material and associated clinical and health data that is stored, processed, and distributed for ongoing and future scientific research.
3 The adjectives 'personalised' and 'precision' have been used interchangeably to popularise what more accurately should be termed pharmogenomic-based medicine (PGx).
4 Priority-setting strategies are discussed in detail in Chapter 3.
5 The global economic process of 'financialisation' is described in Chapter 1.
6 The 'core biopharmaceutical sector' is defined by the UK government as including all busi-nesses involved in 'developing and/or producing their own pharmaceutical products – from small, R&D focused biotechs to Big Pharma' (ONS:2024).
7 The concept of 'governance' in the context of health policy was discussed in detail in Chapter 3.
8 The role of NICE and its HTA process is discussed in detail in Chapter 7.
9 The role of the Quality Outcomes Framework system is discussed in detail in Chapter 7.
10 Lukes' three-dimensional model of power is discussed in relation to the policy process in Chapter 2.

References

Borup, M, Brown, N, Konrad, K and Van Lente, H (2006) The sociology of expectations in science and technology, *Technological Analysis and Strategic Management*, vol. 18, no. 3, 285–298.

Cleary, E, Beierlein, J, Khanuja, N, McNamee, L and Ledley, F (2018) Contribution of NIH funding to new drug approvals 2010–2016, *PNAS*, vol. 115, no. 10, 2329–2334.

Corporate Europe Observatory (2021) *Big Pharma's lobbying firepower in Brussels*. www.corporateeurope.org (accessed 04/2023).

Crinson, I (2021) *The Biomedical Sciences in Society: An Interdisciplinary Perspective*. London. Palgrave Macmillan.

Dearden, N (2023) *Pharmanomics: How Big Pharma Destroys Global Health*. London. Verso Books

Dumit, J (2012) *Drugs for Life: How Pharmaceutical Companies Define Our Health*. Durham & London. Duke University Press.

Edgar, A (2013) The dominance of Big Pharma: power, *Medicine, Health Care and Philosophy*, vol. 16, 295–304.

EFPIA – European Federation of Pharmaceutical Industries and Associations (2022) Pharmaceutical Market Value. www.efpia.eu (accessed 03/24)

Elliott, R, Camacho, E, Campbell, F, Jankovic, D, Martyn St James, M, Kaltenthaler, E, Wong, R, Sculpher, M and Faria, R (2018) *Prevalence and Economic Burden of Medication Errors in the NHS in England*. Sheffield. Policy Research Unit in Economic Evaluation of Health & Care Interventions (EEPRU).

FDA – Federal Food and Drug Administration (2024) *Table of Pharmocogenomic Biomarkers in Drug Labeling*. www.fda.gov (accessed 04/2024).

Fernandez, R and Klinge, T (2020) *The Financialisation of Big Pharma*. Amsterdam, NL. Stichting Onderzoek Multinationale Indernemingem (SOMA).

Ginsburg, G and Philips, K (2018) Precision medicine from science to value. *Health Affairs*, vol. 37, no. 5, 694–701.

Haslem, C, Leaver, A, Murphy, R and Tsitsianis, N (2021) *Assessing the Impact of Shareholder Primacy and Value Extraction*. Productivity Insights Network Blog. Productivityinsightsnetwork.co.uk.

Hawksbee, L, McKee, M and King, L (2022) Don't worry about the drug ndustry's profits when considering a waiver on COVID-19 intellectual property rights, *British Medical Journal*, vol. 376, e067367.

HM Treasury (2005) Public Expenditure 2004–05. Cm 6639. London. The Stationary Office

HM Treasury (2021) *Build Back Better: Our Plan for Growth*. CP 401. London. HM Treasury.

Khoury, M, Bowen, S, Dotson, W, Drzymalla, E, Green, R, Goldstein, R, Kolor, K, Liburb, L, Sperling, L and Bunnell, R (2022) Health equity in the implementation of genomics and precision medicine: a public health imperative, *Genetics in Medicine*, vol. 24, 1630–1639.

Krebs, K and Milani, L (2019) Translating pharmacogenomics into clinical decisions: do not let the perfect be the enemy of the good, *Human Genomics*, vol. 13, 39.

Lukes, S (1974) *Power: A Radical View*. Basingstoke. Macmillan.

Lukes, S (2004) *Power: A Radical View* (2nd Ed). London. Palgrave.

Magavern, E, Daly, A, Gilchrist, A and Hughes, D (2021) Pharmacogenomics spotlight commentary: from the United Kingdom to global populations, *British Journal of Clinical Pharmacology*, vol. 87, 4549–4551.

Moore, D (2021) Pharma companies spend billions more on stock buybacks than developing drugs. *American Prospect*. July 15, 2021.

Naci, H and Forrest, R (2023) *Pharmaceutical Policy in the UK*. London. LSE/The Health Foundation.

NHS Digital (2005) *Prescribing Costs in Hospitals and the Community 2004–05*. https://digital.nhs.uk (accessed 03/24).

NHS Digital (2020) *Prescribing Costs in Hospitals and the Community 2019–20*. https://digital.nhs.uk (accessed 03/24).

NHS England (2020) *Annual Report and Accounts 2019–20*. HC 1027. London. NHS.

NHSBSA – National Health Service Business Services Authority (2023) Prescribing Costs in Hospitals and Community – England 2022–23. https://nhsbsa.nhs.uk (accessed 03/24).

NIH – National Institutes of Health (2024) *News and Events – February 19th*. https://www.allofus.nih.gov (accessed 04/2024).

ONS – Office of National Statistics (2024) *Bioscience and health technology sector statistics 2021 to 2022*. www.ons.gov.uk (accessed 05/2024).

Rafi, I, Crinson, I, Dawes, M, Rafi, D, Pirmohamed, M and Walter, FM (2020) The implementation of pharmacogenomics into UK general practice: a qualitative study exploring barriers, challenges and opportunities, *Journal of Community Genetics*, vol. 11, no. 3, 269–277.

Roden, D, MacLeod, H, Relling, M, Mensah, G, Peterson, J and Van Driest, S (2019) Genomics medicine 2 – pharmacogenomics, *The Lancet*, vol. 394, no. 10197, 521–532.

RPS – Royal Pharmaceutical Society (2014) *New Medicines, Better Medicines, Better Use of Medicines*. London. RPS.

Stark, Z, and 14 other contributing authors (2019) Integrating genomics into healthcare: a global responsibility, *The American Journal of Human Genetics*, vol. 104, no. 1, 13–20.

Sukri, A, Salleh, MZ, Masimirembwa, C and The, LK (2022) A systematic review of the cost-effectiveness of pharmacogenomics in developing countries: implementation challenges, *The Pharmacogenomics Journal*, vol. 22, 147–159.

Swift, C (2022) Personalised future prescribing using pharmacogenomics: a resumé of a joint Royal College of Physicians/British Pharmacological society working party report, *Future Healthcare Journal*, vol. 9, no. 2, 174–178.

Tutton, R (2014) *Genomics and the Reimagining of Personalized Medicine*. Farnham. Ashgate.

Tutton, R (2016) 'Personal genomics and its sociotechnical transformations' in Kumar, D and Chadwick, R (eds) *Genomics and Society*. London. Academic Press. pp 1–20.

UK Biobank (2024) *Why we have sequenced half a million genomes?* https://ukbiobank.ac.uk (accessed 04/2024).

Youssef, E, Kirkdale, C, Wright, D, Guchelaar, H and Thornley, T (2021) Estimating the potential impact of implementing pre-emptive pharmacogenomic testing in primary care across the UK, *British Journal of Clinical Pharmacology*, vol. 87, no. 7, 2907–2925.

Brief reflections on the study of health policy

Health policy analysis is always a dynamic sphere for social and political research, and therefore engaging in the assessment of some new development within a health system can sometimes appear to be like trying to hit a moving target. The real world of health policy decision-making doesn't appear to engender contemplative assessment, but there is an alternative to reductive empiricism and fragmentary understanding. There are identifiable continuities in health policy that can be identified through systematic comparative analysis, these include the rising demand such as the demand for effective and accessible health care provision, and with it the ever-present question of how best to equitably fund these services. Equally, while the role of the national state in health and welfare provision has changed considerably over the decades but is is also clear that reliance on the private market for the equitable as well as effective provision of services is not a realistic option. In order to contextualise these constants of health policy analysis some form of systematic and historical-institutional conceptual framing is required. Some modest examples of this interdisciplinary approach are provided within the pages of this book.

Iain Crinson – September 2024

DOI: 10.4324/9781003564249-15

Index

Printed in the United States
by Baker & Taylor Publisher Services